101

VETERINARY TECHNICIAN
QUESTIONS ANSWERED

Katherine Dobbs, RVT, CVPM, PHR

D1432591

American Animal Hospital Association Press
12575 West Bayaud Avenue
Lakewood, Colorado 80228
800/252-2242 or 303/986-2800
AAHAPress@aahanet.org
www.aahanet.org

Library of Congress Cataloging-in-Publication Data

Dobbs, Katherine.
 101 veterinary technician questions answered / Katherine Dobbs.
 p. cm.
 ISBN 1-58326-106-0 (alk. paper)
   1. Animal health technicians—Handbooks, manuals, etc. 2. Animal health
technology—Handbooks, manuals, etc. I. Title. II. Title: One hundred and one veterinary
technician questions answered. III. Title: One hundred one veterinary technician questions
answered.
 SF774.4.D63 2009
  636.089'0737069—dc22   2009005299
                              CIP

Printed in the United States of America

 9 8 7 6 5 4 3 2 1

Interior design by Elizabeth Lahey.
Cover design by Erin Johnson Design.

DEDICATION

For my family, both human and furry, especially Mary Ann and Katie.

TABLE OF CONTENTS

PREFACE

What compels us to enter the field of veterinary medicine? More importantly, what keeps us here? You may wonder why, when you have been on your feet for ten hours with no lunch break, when you are covered with blood, feces, and vomit, when you have just argued with your boss and you've had to euthanize your favorite patient. Yet you'll wake up the next day, pull on your scrubs, walk through the doors of your practice, and face another day of poop and puppy kisses, high maintenance clients and thankful coworkers, senile cats and wary Rottweilers, all because of your love for this profession.

What began as a love for animals was enhanced by a connection to clients, who share the same bond to their pets as you have to yours. As you immersed yourself in the work to make pets healthier and live longer, you realized that you share this goal with the people toiling beside you, and mutual respect sprouted. Whether you have just attended your first seminar or your hundredth lecture, you have learned to appreciate how versatile and dynamic this profession truly is. You discovered your potential to grow constantly in your knowledge and skills.

The purpose of this publication is to provide you information, resources, and inspiration. When we asked technicians to share their most challenging problems, two thirds of the responses involved career and personal development, and the promotion of our profession. It became obvious that while we feel we have conquered many of the technical skills involved in veterinary technology, it is the issues that appear to be beyond our control that trouble us most. One respondent said, "How do I stay inspired when I'm tired, the clients are driving me nuts, and I would like to push my doctor off a cliff?" There is no doubt you feel this way some days, and need some inspiration too. You may find the inspiration you seek in this book, either in a comment from one of your colleagues or in the form of a practical tip to make your day run more smoothly. One thing is certain: Together, we make a difference every day to the pets in our care, the pet owners who trust us to help, and the professionals that share our desire to pursue this career in veterinary medicine.

Please note that we have used "she" to refer to technicians, veterinarians, and dogs, and we have used "he" to refer to clients, managers, and cats. We simply wanted to avoid an awkward "he or she" sentence construction, and we made this split randomly.

ABOUT THE AUTHOR

Katherine Dobbs, RVT, CVPM, PHR, began her career in veterinary medicine by becoming a registered veterinary technician in 1992. Since that time, her love of animals and the veterinary profession has led her down a path toward practice management and human resources, yet she is never far from her roots as a technician. She has moved into a career of consulting with the intention of helping technicians and all veterinary professionals discover or maintain a career path that is both personally satisfying and professionally successful.

ACKNOWLEDGMENTS

Mentors have been so important in my career. I would like to express my appreciation to Vickie Lawrence, DVM, who showed me how a veterinarian could really be part of a pet's family, and who provided me the opportunity to learn all aspects of veterinary practice while pursuing my veterinary education; and to George Younger, DVM, who inspired excellence at Tomball College during my years in the veterinary technology program, and provided me the education I needed to move forward. Most especially, I am thankful for the guidance of Derek Burney, DVM, PhD, DACVIM, who taught me so much about connecting with clients and with the veterinary team. I am grateful for my years of veterinary experience and opportunity.

This book was made possible by friends and colleagues who share the veterinary technician profession. I am appreciative of those technicians who told us about the greatest challenges in their work, and the technicians who responded to those challenges with lessons to share and inspiration to give. Veterinary technicians are an amazing group of professionals, and you are all appreciated for your accomplishments.

For those who contributed to this book, I thank you[1]:

Alexa Pickles, CVT, Friendship Hospital for Animals, Fort Collins, CO

Alexandra Dashkevicz, BS, BA, RVT, Town and Country Veterinary Services, Manalapan, NJ

Alexis M. Henry, LVT, Animal Health Clinic, Fargo, ND

Alicia Lee, CVT, Cleveland Heights Animal Hospital, Lakeland, FL

Alisha Young, RVT, Spring Meadow Veterinary Clinic, Ashland, OH

Alison Lessard, LVT, Telford, PA

Amanda Henry, CVT, Janesville Animal Medical Center, Janesville, WI

Amber L. Williams, CVT, Berkshire Veterinary Hospital, Pittsfield, MA

Amy Campbell, CVT, VTS (ECC), Tufts Veterinary Emergency Treatment and Specialties, Walpole, MA

Amy Klotz, Douds Veterinary Hospital, Oberlin, OH

Andrea (Andi) Nelsen, CVT, VTS (ECC), Animal Wellness Center of Maple Grove, Maple Grove, MN

Andrea J. Pulzone, CVT, Ark Animal Hospital, Philomath, OR

Anne Matz, RVT

Aylah Skultety, Red Bank Veterinary Hospital, Tinton Falls, NJ

Barbara McCullough, CVT, Russell Veterinary Hospital, P.C., Russell, PA

Becky Ramiz, CVT, MVS, Miami, FL

Beth Finnegan, LVT, Greenbriar Veterinary Referral and Emergency Hospital, Frederick, MD

Beth Galligan, RVT, Kansas State University Veterinary Medical Teaching Hospital, Manhattan, KS

Beth Stawicki, CVT, Raritan Animal Hospital, Edison, NJ

Beverly Baumgartner, LVT, Spencer Springs Animal Hospital, Las Vegas, NV

Blythe M. Swanger, BS, RVT, Broad Ripple Animal Clinic, Indianapolis, IN

Bobbi Jo King, RVT, Elk Grove, CA

Bonnie Loghry, RVT, Yuba College Veterinary Technology Program, Marysville, CA

Bree Bruski, Lextron Animal Health, Billings, MT

Brenda K. Feller, RVT, CVT, VCA, Indianapolis Veterinary Clinic, Indianapolis, IN

Brenna Johnson, CVT, Rochester, MN

Cari Mills, All Pet Emergency Clinic, Evansville, IN

Carl Koop, CVT, Advance Equine Dentistry, Parker, CO

Carol A. Gault, RVT, RLATG, Pfizer Animal Health, Kalamazoo, MI

Caroline Tibbetts, RVT, West Manheim Animal Hospital, Hanover, PA

Catharine Doucette, CVT, Kingston Animal Hospital, Kingston, MA

Cecilia Garza, CVT, RVT, Louisville Family Animal Hospital, Louisville, CO

Chantelle Tebaldi, CVT, Angell Animal Medical Center, Boston, MA

Char Mason, LVT, VTS (ECC), Animal Emergency and Critical Care at The Life Centre, Leesburg, VA

Cheryl Porter, LVT, Fort Hunt Animal Hospital, Alexandria, VA

Christina May Chatham, Arizona Animal Wellness Center, Gilbert, AZ

Christina Mullins, LVT, Kings Veterinary Hospital, Cincinnati, OH

Christine E. Murphy, LVT, Flannery Animal Hospital, New Windsor, NY

Christine M.H. White, CVT, Small Animal Surgical Service, LLC, Wallingford, CT

Christine Schultz, CVT, Burr Ridge Veterinary Clinic, Burr Ridge, IL

Christy Miles, LVT, VTS (ECC), Veterinary Emergency Treatment Service, Charlottesville, VA

Cindi Wyatt, Head Veterinary Technician, Desert Tails Animal Clinic, Scottsdale, AZ

Cindy Dittmar, RVT, Henderson, TX

Cindy Wright, CVT, Mountain View Animal Hospital, Scotrun, PA

Conni L. Bills, LVT, Farmington Veterinary Hospital, Farmington, NY

Crystal Schaeffer, Noahs Animal Hospital, Indianapolis, IN

Dana Fehl, CVT, Duncan Manor Animal Hospital, Allison Park, PA

Danielle Bedard, LVT, Craig Road Animal Hospital, Las Vegas, NV

Danielle K. Simmons, CVT, Abington Veterinary Center, Clarks Summit, PA

Darci L. Harris, CVT, Adobe Veterinary Center, Tucson, AZ

David L., CVT, LVT, Fort Wright Pet Care and Surgical Center, Fort Wright, KY

Dawn Bolka, RVT, BSBA, Hobart Animal Clinic, Hobart, IN

Dawn M. Ellis, CVT, SC Surgical Referral Service, Columbia, SC

Dawn Marie Perault, CVT, Century Animal Clinic, Maplewood, MN

Dawn Terrill, CVT, Veterinary Emergency & Specialty Hospital, South Deerfield, MA

Deb Buttke, RVT, CVT, Prairie Hills Pet Clinic, Milbank, SD

Debbie Kiernan, RVT, Walnut Creek Animal Clinic, Mansfield, TX

Denise DeCarlo, Noahs Brandywine Animal Health Care Center, Greenfield, IN

Denise Lenhart, LVT, Hudson Highlands, Hopewell Junction, NY

Diane Becker, RVT, Animal Medical Hospital, Charlotte, NC

Diane W. Culver, LVT, Stack Veterinary Hospital, Syracuse, NY

Donna Broussard, Preston Royal Animal Clinic, Dallas, TX

Donna J. Johnston, RVT, IWCC, Veterinary Technology, Council Bluffs, IA

Ed Huntley, CVT, Brookside Veterinary Hospital, Bridgeport, CT

Elizabeth J. Hughes, CVT, Falls Road Veterinary Hospital, Potomac, MD

Elizabeth M. Johnson-Rhodes, RVT, CCRA, VCA, Woodland South Animal Hospital and Canine Rehabilitation Center, Tulsa, OK

Elizabeth Olvera, RVT, Defiance, OH

Elizabeth Warren, RVT, Austin, TX

Erika Ervin, BS, CVT, Oakhurst Veterinary Hospital, Oakhurst, NJ

Fiona M. Christie, RVT, Akron, OH

Francine Dermer, LVT, Springfield Veterinary Center, Glen Allen, VA

Gail Finkelstein, LVT, Roundhill Animal Hospital, Zephyr Cove, NV

Gerianne Holzman, CVT, VTS (Dentistry), Veterinary Medical Teaching Hospital, Madison, WI

Gina Falish, CVT, Animal Emergency and Treatment Center, Grayslake, IL

Gina Harrison, RVT, Bright Eyes & Bushy Tails Veterinary Hospital, Iowa City, IA

Goksun Deniz, LVT, Hoboken, NJ

Heather Bowen, CVT, Buzzards Bay Veterinary Associates, Buzzards Bay, MA

Heidi Reinhardt, CVT, Bobtown Pet Clinic, Roberts, WI

Helen R. DeWitt, CVT, Grayslake Animal Hospital, Grayslake, IL

I. Sean Seelhoff, LVT, Baker College of Muskegon, Muskegon, MI

Jamie Kavan, LVT, ToMorrow's Veterinary Care, Waverly, NE

Janice W. Hayes, BS, RVT, Cohutta Animal Clinic, Blue Ridge, GA

Jasmine J. Johnsen, VT, CVA, Avian and Feline Hospital, Camp Hill, PA

Jasminne Nash, RVT, Riverstone Animal Hospital, Canton, GA

Jennifer Henze, LVT, Glove Cities Veterinary Hospital, P.C., Gloversville, NY

Jennifer Klotch, RVT, County of San Diego Animal Services, San Diego, CA

Jennifer Leo, CVT, Animal Hospital of Ashwaubenon, Green Bay, WI

Jennifer S. Limon, RVT, Delgado Community College, Covington, LA

Jessica Maloy, LVT, Animal Health Center, Enterprise, AL

Jessica Pascal, CVT, Veterinary Surgical and Diagnostic Specialists, Clarksburg, NJ

Jill Betz, LVT, Red Cedar Animal Hospital PC, Okemos, MI

Jill Foster, RVT, Indian Hills Animal Clinic, Wichita, KS

JoAnn Gammon, CVT, Animal Hospital, Longmont, CO

Joanne Light, LVT, Paradise Pet Hospital, Las Vegas, NV

Jodean Hipke, CVT, Peshtigo Veterinary Service, Peshtigo, WI

Joseph D'Abbraccio, LVT, Monhagen Veterinary Hospital, Middletown, NY

Karen Eckhoff, RVT, San Diego Humane Society and SPCA, San Diego, CA

Karen Lynn Moes, Ottawa Animal Hospital, Holland, MI

Katelyn Little, CVT, Intown Veterinary Group, Woburn, MA

Kathy Cetron, CVT, Home Veterinary Service, Belford, NJ

Kathy Daily, RVT, El Dorado Animal Clinic, El Dorado, KS

Kathy Elbel, LVT, Lee's Summit Animal Hospital, PC, Lee's Summit, MO

Kathy Simpson, BBA, RVT, Albuquerque Cat Clinic, Albuquerque, NM

Kellie Bartett, RVT, LVT, SAMP, Advanced Care Animal Clinic, Arlington, WA

Kendell Brichacek, LVT, Bar-S Veterinary Clinic, David City, NE

Kerry Howard, CVT, Verona Veterinary Medical Service S.C., Verona, WI

Kim Buethe, LVT, Best Care Pet Hospital, Omaha, NE

Kim Innes, CVT, All County Animal Hospital, Brooksville, FL

Kim M. Novick, CVT, Veterinary Learning Systems, Yardley, PA

Kimberley A. Tidball, CVT, Bayleaf Veterinary Hospital, Raleigh, NC

Kristin P. Coppola, CVT, Phoenix Veterinary Hospital, Wayland, MA

Krystal Sobrino, CVT, LVT, All Pets Animal Hospital, Peoria, AZ

Laura K. Frazier, BA, AAT, RVT, Highland Animal Hospital, Augusta, GA

Lauren Blue, BS, Garden Creek Pet Clinic, Greensboro, NC

Leah Erickson, CVT, Cannon Valley Veterinary Clinic, Northfield, MN

Lee Apua'latl, CVT, Riverbend Animal Hospital, Hadley, MA

Lewanne E. Hunt Sharp, BA, RVT, VTS (ECC), Mesa Community College Veterinary Technology Program, Mesa, AZ

Linda Hennessy, RVT, Diablo View Veterinary Hospital, Pleasant Hill, CA

Linda Merrill, LVT, VTS (SAIM), Seattle Veterinary Associates, Seattle, WA

Linda Myers, CVT, Perkiomen Animal Hospital, Palm, PA

Lindsay Y. Feerrar, CVT, Neffsville Veterinary Clinic, and Lancaster Career and Technology Center, Lancaster, PA

Lisa Cothran, Vet Pets Animal Hospital, Cordova, TN

Lisa Paquette, Asheville Buncombe Technical Community College, Asheville, NC

Lisa Redington, LVT, Mobile Animal Clinic, Omaha, NE

Lisa Tucker, RVT, Forsyth Animal Hospital, Cumming, GA

Liz Culver, CVT, All Creatures Veterinary Hospital, Coventry, CT

Liza Wysong Rudolph, LVT, Metropolitan Veterinary Associates, Valley Forge, PA

Lyndi M. Watson, LVT, Pebble Creek Animal and Bird Hospital, Tampa, FL

Lynn A. Loper, CVT, Stafford Veterinary Hospital, Manahawkin, NJ

Lynn Presnell, RVT, Doc-Side Veterinary Medical Center, Baltimore, MD

M. Nicole Petrovich, RVT, Carlsbad Animal Hospital, Carlsbad, CA

Margot Williams, RVT, Oakland Animal Hospital, Oakland, NJ

Marisa Rhyne, RVT, VTS (ECC), Veterinary Specialists of North Texas, Dallas, TX

Marjorie DeMeyere, LVT, Maple Veterinary Hospital, Troy, MI

Mark Horton, CVT, Veterinary Surgical Services, Englewood, CO

Mark L. Hoag, LVT, Colonie Animal Hospital, Albany, NY

Mary Catherine Costello, CVT, Shoreview North Oaks Animal Hospital, Shoreview, MN

Mary Grace G. Phillips, RVT, Great Lakes Veterinary Specialists, Bedford Hts., OH

Mary M. Bramer, LVT, Burnt Hills Veterinary Hospital, Burnt Hills, NY

Mary Matthews, CVT, Lantana-Atlantis Animal Hospital, Lantana, FL

Maureen Hagen, LVT, Town Center Veterinary Associates, Howell, MI

Maxine Hladky, LVT, VCA Black Mountain Animal Hospital, Henderson, NV

Megan Licht, LVT, Transit Animal Hospital, Depew, NY

Melissa J. Sloss, LVT, RVT, Auburn University Small Animal Teaching Hospital, Auburn, AL

Melissa Siekaniec, CVT, VTS (ECC), Florida Veterinary Specialists, Tampa, FL

Melody Quammen, CVT, San Juan Veterinary Clinic, Montrose, CO

Melody Thompson, RVT, Equine Medical Associates, Edmond, OK

Michele Guzik-Mosher, CVT, Center for Animal Referral & Emergency Services, Langhorne, PA

Michele L. Murphy, LVT, CVT, Woodland Animal Clinic, DeLand, FL

Michele Laughlin, CVT, Parker Center Animal Clinic, Parker, CO

Michelle Brevard, CVT, Brooklyn Veterinary Clinic, Castle Rock, CO

Michelle Keith, LVT, Westgate Veterinary Hospital, Enterprise, AL

Michelle Lewis, CVT, Magic Valley Veterinary Hospital, Twin Falls, ID

Michelle Miller, BS, CVT, University of Minnesota, Veterinary Medical Center, St. Paul, MN

Michelle Sledge, LVT, Crestwood Veterinary Hospital, Crestwood, KY

Mindy Bough, CVT, ASPCA Midwest Office, Urbana, IL

Misty Woolf, RVT, Colonial Terrace Animal Hospital, Dubuque, IA

Monique Pierpont, Harmony Animal Hospital, Jupiter, FL

Nancy A. Miller, RVT, Kimberly Crest Veterinary Hospital, Davenport, IA

Nancy A. Roth, BS, RVT, SRA, Eureka Veterinary Clinic, Eureka, MO

Nancy K. Robinson, RVT, LVT, Central Carolina Community College, Sanford, NC

Natalie Wilson Hosp, CVT, RDH, Shaffer Animal Hospital, Oviedo, FL

Nicole Tanton, LVT, West Mountain Animal Hospital, Bennington, VT

Nicole Tougas, LVT, Norfolk SPCA Veterinary Hospital, Norfolk, VA

Pamela S. Morosky, RVT, Minerva Veterinary Clinic, Minerva, OH

Pamella A. McCoy, RVT, Advanced Care Animal Clinic, Arlington, WA

Peg L. Phillips, RVT, CVT, Fostoria Animal Hospital, Hoyrtville, OH

R.M. (Ann) Gillespie, RVT, Fort Valley State University, Fort Valley, GA

Rebecca A. Klahn-Schwartz, CVT, Cedar Grove Veterinary Services, Cedar Grove, WI

Rebecca Rose, CVT, Red Valley Rose Consulting, Gunnison, CO

Rene Scalf, CVT, VTS (ECC, SAIM), Colorado State University Veterinary Teaching Hospital, Fort Collins, CO

Rhonda Baillargeon, LVT, Turner Veterinary Service, Turner, ME

Rosanne Beauchemin, LVT, Spring Valley Animal Hospital, Monsey, NY

Rose Marie A. Binder, LVT, NVA, Rochester Veterinary Hospital, Rochester Hills, MI

Sally Gosselin, CVT, Salmon Brook Veterinary Hospital, Granby, CT

Samantha Rowland, LVT, Veterinary Emergency Treatment Service, Charlottesville, VA

Sandra Hering, CVT, Pioneer Veterinary Clinic, Corvallis, OR

Sandra K. Black, RVT, Bigger Road Veterinary Clinic, Kettering, OH

Sara James, LVT, Twin Lakes Veterinary Hospital, Federal Way, WA

Sarah Gardner, CVT, The Animal Hospital of Barrington, Barrington, NH

Sarah Wright, CVT, Bellevue Animal Clinic, Little Rock, AR

SGT Erin Reymann, CVT, LVT, Fort Gordon Veterinary Treatment Facility, Fort Gordon, GA

Sharon Garland, LVT, Meadowridge Veterinary Hospital, Groton, NY

Sharon Klingler, RVT, VTS (Anesthesia), All About Pets, Whitesboro, TX

Sharon M. Johnston, LVT, VTS (Anesthesia)

Shelly Strusz, CVT, Zumbrota Veterinary Clinic, Zumbrota, MN

Shelly, Chestnut Street Animal Hospital, Needham, MA

Stephanie J. Getz, CVT, Southampton, PA

Stephanie Taylor, LVT, Centreville Animal Hospital, Centreville, PA

Suesan Larsen, RVT, Mother Lode Veterinary Hospital, Grass Valley, CA

Sunni Willis, CVT, North Main Street Veterinary Clinic, Brockton, MA

Susan Erhardt, LVT, Baring Blvd. Animal Hospital, Sparks, NV

Susan Evans, CVT, South Wilton Veterinary Group, Wilton, CT

Susan Holland, LVT, VTS (Anesthesia), Animal Cancer and Imaging Center, Canton, MI

Suzanne Wickham, RVT, Heartwood Animal Hospital, Youngsville, NC

Suzy Kafuman, RVT, Stautzenberger College, Brecksville, OH

Tammy S. Aylward, LVT, Animal Skin and Allergy Clinic, Lynnwood, WA

Taryn Singleton, LVT, Sycamore Veterinary Hospital, Midlothian, VA

Teresa A. Marcolini, CVT, Bright Cross Animal Clinic, Venice, FL

Theresa Miresse, CVT, Wisconsin Veterinary Referral Center, Waukesha, WI

Tim Wells, LVT, Shawnee Animal Clinic, Inc., Portsmouth, OH

Tina Microutsicos, BS, CVT, Princeton Animal Hospital, Princeton, NJ

Toni Andersen, RVT, Belmont Shore Veterinary Hospital, Long Beach, CA

Tosha Mallery, CVT, Sun City Animal Hospital, Sun City, AZ

Tracey Nowers, CVT, Gardner Animal Care Center, Gardner, MA

Tricia Wallace, LVT, Michigan Veterinary Specialists, Southfield, MI

V. A. Schroeder, RVT, RLATG, University of Notre Dame, Notre Dame, IN

Vicki Jones, RVT, Emporia Veterinary Hospital, Emporia, KS

Victoria Kasel, CVT, Welcome All Pets Veterinary Care, Queen Creek, AZ

Virginia R. Crossett, RVT, Louisville Zoological Gardens, Louisville, KY

[1]Please note that these names were copied directly from the responses the technicians provided. We did correct the obvious mistakes in names of respondents and hospitals. Also, some contributors remained anonymous, and so they are not listed here.

1

CAREER DEVELOPMENT

Most of you recognize that being a veterinary technician is not just a job, it is a career and you are a professional. Every profession has its challenges, as does veterinary technology. We identified three concerns shared by many of us: finding good experienced technicians, keeping good technicians happy, and being paid what we are worth. These issues do not stand alone; they build on each other. The solution to one will lead to solving the others. If we can get paid well, we'll stay in the profession longer and be happier, creating a more experienced workforce. As we become more experienced, we are likely to be paid more and become more satisfied in a career where constant learning can invigorate and inspire us. Lastly, if we can be happy in our jobs we will be a more positive influence on our practice, deserve to get paid a higher wage, and stay in the profession longer.

Where do we start? With a good job, and a chance to make a difference and grow personally and professionally.

How do I find out what areas in the job market are available to a veterinary technician?

Keep your eyes open! You can search both inside and outside of veterinary medicine resources. Online sources such as Craigslist and Monster Jobs can lead you to some interesting job openings for people with our backgrounds. Within the veterinary world, there are online sources such as the Veterinary Support Personnel Network (VSPN) and VetMedTeam. Numerous veterinary publications provide employment information, including *Veterinary Technician Journal,* the *NAVTA Journal,* and *Veterinary Practice News.*

Make it a habit to scan the classified ad sections of these journals, even when you're not actively looking for a new job. It is especially helpful to read the biographies of other veterinary technicians to see what type of careers they have pursued. You can learn about the opportunities that have led them down their career paths, and decide if their final destination is where you might like to be some day.

The national, state, and local technician associations can be a good source for learning about job options. There are other sources that you may not have considered, such as your local or state veterinary technology program(s) and veterinary schools.

How about those sales representatives who come through your practice? They may know of interesting options both within their company and the local or regional community they travel every day. Finally, talk to other technicians. While attending seminars and lectures with other technicians, talk about what you do and where you work. Visit the exhibit hall and notice career options in the military or in veterinary industry, such as pet insurance providers, software and technology companies, pharmaceutical companies, pet food manufacturers, and pet supply distributors. You may discover some interesting career paths. You may be able to ask questions at the same time. These recommended resources can help you locate opportunities in companion animal medicine, and beyond.

RESOURCES
AnimalJobs.com, www.animaljobs.com

CareerBuilder.com, www.careerbuilder.com

Career Choices for Veterinary Technicians: Opportunities for Animal Lovers, by Rebecca
  Rose, CVT, and Carin Smith, DVM (AAHA Press 2009)

CareerSniff, www.careersniff.com

CraigsList, www.craigslist.org/about/sites

iHireVeterinary, www.ihireveterinary.com

JobConnect.com, www.jobconnect.com

Monster, www.monster.com

National Association of Veterinary Technicians in America, www.navta.net

NAVTA Journal, www.navta.net

Veterinary Career Network, www.veterinarycareernetwork.com

Veterinary Information Network, www.vin.com

Veterinary Management Groups, www.findvmgjobs.com

Veterinary Practice News, www.veterinarypracticenews.com

Veterinary Support Personnel Network, www.vspn.org, vetquest.com

Veterinary Technician Journal, www.vettechjournal.com

Veterinary Technicians and Assistants Resource Center, www.vtarc.com

VetMedTeam, www.vetmedteam.com

WhereTechsConnect.com, www.wheretechsconnect.com

Yahoo! Hotjobs, www.hotjobs.yahoo.com

How do I find a great clinic to work at, and how do I know when I've found a great clinic?

Finding a great clinic to work at is all about the interview process. We typically think of an interview as an opportunity for the employer to see if they want to choose us. Actually, it is just as important to determine if this job would be the best fit for us. Go into an interview determined to sell yourself, but also be prepared to conduct an interview of your own.

Prior to the interview, research the facility as much as possible. Examine their Web site, paying particular attention to their stated mission, the philosophy they demonstrate, the services they provide, and the type of facility.

When applying for the position, take your résumé (with a tailored cover letter) to the facility in person, so you can examine the public areas and obtain any printed material available for client education. This is particularly important if the practice does not have a Web site.

Read all of these materials, and write down several questions that are important to you and your job satisfaction. Ask these questions during the interview. You may need to inquire about scheduling and job duties; but remember to consider questions of a deeper nature. You may want to ask about management philosophy, medical ethics, and staff communication and morale. Find out how the clinic recognizes and rewards credentialed technicians with continuing education opportunities, how they educate the public regarding the importance of credentialed technicians on the team, and what promotion opportunities exist for technicians. You may need to evaluate a few hospitals, or conduct many interviews, to find the right fit for you.

So, once you've accepted a position, how do you know if you've found a great clinic? First of all, observe the practice at work and see if they live up to their own stated mission or values. Veterinary medicine is a profession that cares for animals, but works through people to provide that care. A good clinic focuses on the client/pet relationship and how it relates to their hospital, and provides excellent, personal service to its clients and patients. The people who work at the practice and the loyal clientele who visit make the clinic a wonderful place to work.

The best teams have active communication between staff members, including veterinarians who actively seek opinions from the technical staff who are observing the patients. A good team works together without distrust or tension between the front and back staff. Everyone on the staff works toward the goal of repeat clients who are satisfied that their pets are getting the quality care they deserve.

How do I find my niche within a hospital environment?

Once you have found a great clinic, you need to carve out your own niche within that practice. Each person has a unique role on the team; even when two people are in the same position they fill different roles.

The best way to identify your niche is to discover what you are passionate about and pursue that area of interest. If your employer utilizes cross training, use this time to try many different jobs within the practice—for example, surgery, laboratory, appointments, medical record keeping, or client education. This may be possible during your training period. Most practices incorporate cross training at this time so that technicians learn the big picture of the work flow. If cross training is not an option, let your supervisor and colleagues know that you are willing to take shifts in different areas when other employees are on vacation. If you try something new and think you like it, try it again at the next opportunity. If your heart feels excited about coming back to it, then you've found the right spot! Even if you cannot be in that position full-time right away, inform your supervisor of your interest and you may be the next one to fill that spot when it opens. When you've found the right place for yourself, your enthusiasm will become contagious and your coworkers will soon associate you with your passion. Then you will become the in-house expert or go-to person.

What am I worth, for the job I do?
How do I know if I'm getting paid fairly in comparison to technicians at other clinics?

These are two very different questions. First, what you are worth depends on the job that you do. In other words, you need to consider what tasks you perform, how well you perform them, and the difference you make in the practice with regard to client service, patient care, team morale, and practice profitability. That is a personal question that only you can answer, with the help of your supervisor or manager.

The second question involves wage comparison, and there are resources both within and outside of the veterinary profession that can provide this data. Many state government Web sites have a competitive wage resource for that state based on region. The Department of Labor also has statistics available. Within the veterinary profession, look to AAHA, NAVTA, and VHMA surveys to help you compare wages.

There is more to consider than just your hourly wage. Benefits are another part of the compensation package that is often overlooked. Your practice may provide you with this information, or you may need to calculate it yourself. The investment a practice has made in your employment includes legal financial requirements such as social security benefits and workers' compensation insurance. Other, more direct benefits are easier to calculate. These can include continuing education allowance, uniform provisions, paid time off, employee pet and product discounts, and bonuses or gifts.

As you digest these figures, you need to realize that many factors affect wages and benefits. The first of these factors are statistics such as location within the United States, years of experience, type of education, and even the number of hours regularly worked. There are also factors that are more difficult to put into numbers, such as amount of authority and level of responsibility, type of duties assigned and overall workload, increases in skills or knowledge, and overall worth to the practice. Attitude also counts, and a better attitude should be paid better than a poor one.

RESOURCES
American Animal Hospital Association, www.aahanet.org

Department of Labor, www.online.onetcenter.org/link/summary/29-
    2056.00#WagesEmployment
National Association of Veterinary Technicians in America, www.navta.net
Veterinary Hospital Managers Association, www.vhma.org

How do I make myself a more valuable asset to the practice?

You can increase your value to the practice in order to gain more job satisfaction, higher pay, or a promotion you desire. First, demonstrate your knowledge and your continual pursuit to learn more. Veterinary medicine is not a stagnant field; it continues to grow and change every year with new advances in medications, treatments, equipment, and perspectives. Attend as many continuing education classes as possible. This may require you to spend money on your professional advancement beyond any allowance provided by your practice (if there is one). Bring your knowledge back to your practice and teach others with presentations, reports, or demonstrations. As you learn more about the medical care that is offered by your practice, you become more comfortable with the subject or product.

Clients will sense your confidence and will trust your recommendations. Building good client relationships is essential. We are entrusted with people's pets because they feel comfortable with us. With this personal relationship intact, even when mistakes are made or money is tight, clients will return to your practice instead of going elsewhere. This affects the profitability of the practice and your value can be measured in dollars and cents.

A practice that fully utilizes its technicians will pull ahead. When you do your job well, veterinarians are free to do what only they can do: diagnose, prescribe, and perform surgeries. These are the tasks that directly result in income for the practice and allow the team to see more patients.

Motivation and initiative are valuable traits. If you see something that needs to be done, do it without being asked. If something is wrong, fix it. Be proactive and you will be noticed.

Your relationships with coworkers are also important. When you focus more on team accomplishments and less on your own needs, you increase your value to the practice.

Last, a good attitude toward yourself and your profession is essential. If you believe in educating yourself and others, can keep yourself and your colleagues motivated, and provide leadership or direction within your practice or group, then you become invaluable to your practice.

The question was asked, "How can I make a difference to my practice, when I am "just a technician?" The answer, unfortunately, is that you will never make a difference if you feel you are "just" a technician. When you realize that you are a skilled, knowledgeable, important, and respected member of the pet healthcare team, then you can make all the difference you desire.

How do I ask for a raise, and get the raise I deserve?

We've just seen how you can increase your worth or value to the practice. So before you ask for a raise, be sure you can answer the second part of that question: Do you deserve it? Are you worthy of a raise? If you can answer *yes,* then you need to convince your practice owner or manager. Do not assume they have kept a running tally of all your accomplishments. If your practice is using a self-evaluation process during performance evaluations, this is your opportunity to brag. If not, or if you are inclined to ask for a raise that is not in conjunction with your routine evaluation, then you need to create a brag list.

Many practices are leaving behind the concept of annual raises across the board. They no longer reward employees with a raise just because they have survived another year with the practice. Instead, they want to know what you have contributed over the last year.

Describe your experience and expertise, and the skills and knowledge you have brought to the practice. Discuss how you have helped the practice to save money, and how you have improved work flow by helping the doctors stay on schedule. Tell your employer how you have worked well with your teammates. Demonstrate that you came to work consistently and on time. Discuss how you have provided exceptional patient care.

When listing your continuing education accomplishments, remember to include seminars and lectures, online courses and journal subscriptions, and in-house presentations that you attended and taught yourself.

The management also wants to know how you intend to keep contributing in new ways, when and if you receive the raise you are asking for. Focus on the future, and what accomplishments you plan to achieve next. This requires you to be creative, and think forward. Can you help in an additional area that could benefit from your expertise or experience? Are there new ways to help with inventory, improve the training program, or create client education materials?

You should also revisit the practice's mission or vision, and see how you can help the practice reach that goal. If one goal is excellent client service, develop new ways to reach out and form relationships with your pet owners. If your practice states that they will stay on the cutting edge of technology, then include advanced topics in your continuing education attendance and report back to the practice leaders. While you are bragging about your personal accomplishments, be sure to turn the perspective around to how you have helped the team and the practice, and how your accomplishments have benefited the clients and patients. Ask for a raise, but also explain why you're worth it.

How do I get a promotion?

If you want to keep doing the exact same job and your current duties, then you might continue to receive the same pay. If you're ready to take your career to the next level, perhaps a promotion is in your future. Be sure to voice your desire for a promotion to your employer. Do not assume that your employer knows where you want to be in a year, three years, or ten years. This is a good conversation to have during your performance evaluation, but it can occur at any point during the year.

To be worthy of a promotion, you must exceed your current job expectations. You may be helping in additional areas, taking on projects beyond your normal daily activities, or making suggestions that affect the entire team or practice. Many of the strategies you use to increase your value to the practice can earn you a promotion, because valuable employees are the first chosen for promotions. Expanding your knowledge and being proactive are important for a raise or a promotion. Technicians who are valuable also lead by example. That leadership role may lead to a promotion and a position of more authority or responsibility.

There are times when obtaining a promotion means creating a brand new position within your practice. If your organization doesn't appear to have many rungs on its career ladder, you may think that it is impossible to move upward.

Instead of lamenting over this short stepladder, start identifying what the practice needs and how you might be able to help. As you identify problems within the practice, offer solutions or suggestions for improvement. For example, your practice may benefit from a technician supervisor position that is not in existence now. Describe how this position could improve the quality of care for patients, reduce the workload for the practice manager or owner, or create a leadership role on the floor, working beside the technicians on a daily basis. Perhaps your interest lies in inventory, and you can envision an inventory supervisor position where you monitor needs, place orders, reconcile paperwork, and research best prices and new products. If marketing is your niche, develop the idea for a marketing assistant position in which you research local competition and opportunities, develop promotional brochures and products, produce press releases, and organize community events. If you can visualize the creation of a new position within the practice, outline your ideas and you may find yourself creating and filling a brand new position.

How can I prepare for a position in management?

If you want to move your career up the ladder, then the promotion you seek may involve a management position, or at least additional authority or responsibilities. Whether you are interested in a supervisory position or have your eyes set on an upper management position, in your current position as a technician you can accelerate your career by gaining a basic understanding of management concepts and skills. Many technicians advance to the top of their leadership team by taking on projects that allow them to learn the inner workings of the business. While you continue to work with your technician colleagues, also work closely with others such as doctors, receptionists, and client service representatives to understand their daily tasks and skills and hear the suggestions they offer. Your goal is to learn about all aspects of the veterinary practice and how it operates. It is also to show the entire team that you can assume a leadership role beyond your original group of technicians. You must earn the respect of the entire team in order to lead.

Resources for learning veterinary management are numerous. There are many veterinary journals that contain management education, including *Trends Magazine, Veterinary Economics, Firstline, Veterinary Technician Journal,* and *Veterinary Practice News.* The text *Practice Makes Perfect* is a good basic starting point for topics including inventory management, marketing, and human resources. Online courses in management include those offered by VSPN and VetMedTeam. If you learn better in person and have the opportunity, many of the regional and national seminars are offering basic management tracks.

Outside of the veterinary industry, much can be learned from the "human" business world. Topics of value include leadership, active listening, team synergy, and communication styles and techniques.

All of this "book learning" is important and provides a stable foundation, but the best teacher is a leader you respect within your own practice. When you're considering a move to management or want to learn more about basic management, express this desire to a respected leader and ask that person to be your mentor. Offer your assistance with projects that can help you learn more. Most managers will admit that they learned more from their mistakes than from books, so let them teach you so you can avoid those same mistakes!

There is no substitute for on-the-job experience. At the same time, every team and every individual is so different that flexibility and the ability to think on the spot are vital. Learn as much as you can about the duties of a supervisor or manager, but also educate yourself on the mind-set and perspective that are required by a practice leader.

RESOURCES
Blackwell's Five-Minute Veterinary Practice Management Consult, by Lowell Ackerman, DVM, DACVD, MBA, MPA (Blackwell Publishing 2007)
Practice Made Perfect, by Marsha L. Heinke, DVM, EA, CPA, CVPM; and John B. McCarthy, DVM, MBA (AAHA Press 2001)
Team Satisfaction Pays, by Carin A. Smith, DVM (Smith Veterinary Services 2008)
Trends Magazine, www.aahanet.org
Veterinary Economics and *Firstline,* www.dvm360.com
Veterinary Practice News, www.veterinarypracticenews.com
Veterinary Technician Journal, www.vettechjournal.com

COURSES
Veterinary Hospital Management Certificate, www.spcollege.edu/bachelors/vtech_certificates.php?program=vtech
Veterinary Leadership Academy, www.aahanet.org/education/index.aspx
Veterinary Management Institute, www.aahanet.org/education/index.aspx
Veterinary Management School Levels One and Two, www.aahanet.org/education/index.aspx
Veterinary Support Personnel Network, www.vspn.org
VetMedTeam, www.vetmedteam.com
VMC School of Veterinary Practice Management, www.vmc-inc.com/vmc_school.html

How do I determine if the pay differential is worth seeking technician specialization?

There are many opportunities for you to expand your career. As a technician, you can become specialized in a particular field. To date, there are five academies available to credentialed technicians for specialization: emergency and critical care, anesthesia, dentistry, internal medicine (cardiology, oncology, small animal and large animal internal medicine), and behavior. More academies are being established, including clinical practice and surgery, and the internal medicine academy intends to add the neurology subspecialty as well.

There are many reasons you may desire veterinary technician specialist (VTS) credentials, and the pay differential may certainly be one of them. If you are drawn toward one of the specialization fields, it is important to analyze your current practice and where you will fit in after obtaining your VTS. Is this field an area that the practice intends to move toward; for example, do they want to expand their dental services or open a twenty-four-hour emergency service? If so, your new credentials will benefit the hospital and they may have incentive to pay you a higher wage. Yet, while it's important to understand the potential impact on your paycheck, you are probably motivated by more than just this imagined dollar amount. There is also a personal and professional satisfaction to be gained by specializing in an area of interest, and the pay differential may be the least important factor on your list. It is important to realize this, particularly if your practice is emotionally supportive but cannot financially support your goals. If the pay increase is important to you, and your practice cannot utilize or compensate your additional skills and knowledge, you may choose to move on to a different practice. In the end, the decision must involve the numbers, but it should also involve the opportunity to practice your profession at the highest level possible, share your knowledge and skills with others, and open up future career options.

How do I ask my practice to help me become certified as a veterinary specialist?

You need to tell your employer about the specific benefits of having a technician specialist on staff and the improvements you can bring to the practice. Your specialty skills and knowledge may assist the practice in expanding into other areas such as dentistry or behavior. Your skills could also help provide advanced patient care, such as anesthesia or emergency and critical care. Your specialization may allow the doctors to spend more time with their tasks and clients. As the community and clientele become aware of your technician specialty status, it elevates the practice's reputation.

Demonstrate your sincere interest in this specialty. Show initiative by pointing out the continuing education you have obtained to help you make your decision. Visit the Web site of the VTS academy that you want to explore. Obtain the list of prerequisites to share with your leadership team. The practice needs to be willing to give you the opportunity to collect a case log, research specific patients for your case reports, and schedule your time off so that you can obtain the required continuing education hours. The practice leaders may also want to meet with the practice's medical team to discuss what type of work you will be doing in preparation for your VTS. The team will want to know how they are expected to support you in your education.

When it comes to financial assistance, there are requests you can make or offers the practice may extend to support your journey. This can include allotting or increasing your continuing education funds, assisting with the examination fees, or paying the travel expenses to take the examination. There are even long-term arrangements that can benefit both the practice and the technician. The practice could pay for your education in return for a contracted period of employment once you have attained your credentials. If your specialization does not fit the goals of your current practice, you may need to consider a new employer at some point. It's better to know this going into the commitment rather than later. In the end, specialization needs to be a personal as well as a professional goal for any technician.

RESOURCES
Academy of Internal Medicine for Veterinary Technicians (AIMVT), www.aimvt.com
Academy of Veterinary Behavior Technicians (AVBT), www.svbt.org
Academy of Veterinary Dental Technicians (AVDT), www.avdt.us
Academy of Veterinary Emergency and Critical Care Technicians (AVECCT), www.avecct.org
Academy of Veterinary Technician Anesthetists (AVTA), www.avta-vts.org

How do I recession-proof my job?

It has been said that veterinary medicine is a recession-proof industry, but there may be times when the nation's economy challenges this theory. During periods when people have to analyze every expense, you can expect that their pet care costs will come under scrutiny. Although for a majority of pet owners their pets are their family, some of them may have to choose between putting food on the table in front of their human children and filling up the dog's food bowl. Preventive health care for pets may be put on hold, or delayed indefinitely. This may mean more pets will become sick, and sick pets may wait longer to be taken to the veterinarian. When families of sick or injured pets are forced to make a decision on costly diagnostics and treatment, they may choose euthanasia more often than in the past. This will ultimately affect the practice's profitability, and could affect your position on the payroll. Does this mean you are simply a victim of the circumstances befalling your practice? Yes and no. The best way to recession-proof your job is to never take it for granted and to recognize that veterinary medicine is a business. What you do affects the bottom line every day, during the good and bad times. During difficult times, your practice may need to make some uncomfortable and unpopular decisions regarding employee hours, benefits, and staffing. Prove your value to the practice through your performance, commitment to teamwork, and ability to both reduce expenses and generate revenue. If you are one of the top-level employees, one of the superstars, then you may be able to avoid having your hours cut back, or worse, being laid off.

You would be wise to do your best to keep your morale up, and the morale of the team. Talk about what is happening, but in a positive light—what can *we* do to help? How can we help turn this around for our practice? Client service should always be a priority, but when times are tough, you need to focus even more on creating and maintaining strong client relationships. During these slow periods you and the team have more time on your hands to deliver exceptional service. If there is downtime available, use it productively and demonstrate that you are staying busy in constructive ways. Projects that have been put off during busier times can now be accomplished. The team can brainstorm projects that could reduce expenses and increase revenue. If everyone can pitch in and weather the storm, you may come through a little wet but still on the ship.

2

AVOIDING BURNOUT

How do you define yourself? Yes, you are a technician, but you are many other things at the same time. Perhaps you are a spouse to someone waiting at home. Perhaps you are a parent who has made sacrifices for your family and your career. Certainly you are the son or daughter of parents who infused you with genetic or environmental characteristics. Of course you are also a friend to those who fill your life with laughter and love. Being a technician does not define you; it is part of the total package. Yet it is easy to let this amazing, rewarding, challenging, frustrating, fulfilling career take control of our lives and lead us to a one-dimensional existence. How do you retain the person you are, while doing the work you love? More importantly, how do you continue to do the work you love despite its challenges and frustrations? Burnout affects veterinary technicians individually, and the profession as a whole. Yet there are ways to continue being the person you are, and the technician you love to be, while staying in this fulfilling career.

How do I keep calm
when a day is particularly crazy?

If you have survived any time at all in a veterinary practice, then you probably thrive in a fast-paced, often hectic, environment. Yet even the best of us can become frazzled at times. Before you lose control, which would not be a good career move, stop and take a deep breath. First you have to realize that you can only do one thing at a time. Even when we talk about multi-tasking, you are actually dividing your attention among many tasks that are happening simultaneously. So prioritize what needs to be done. You often know which patients, clients, or coworkers need your most immediate attention. During the crazy moments, you have to step back and visualize the big picture to see where to head next.

It's also important for you to stay tuned to your own emotional and physical well-being. This includes taking a lunch break and frequent short breaks to give you time to regroup and recharge. Get out of the building during lunch, have a picnic in a nearby park, or stroll around the neighborhood listening to your favorite music or to the birds in the trees. If it's been a rough day for the entire team, offer to make a run to pick up refreshments or order pizza for everyone who wants to pitch in. Let go of the stress sometimes by enjoying a joke or a sudden burst of song (preferably when there is not a client in the treatment area). It is no surprise that technicians have a sense of humor and are easily amused: It helps us to diffuse the stress that we face daily. Music is a powerful way to keep spirits high. Radios can be played softly, but changed often according to the team on duty. CDs can be used to elicit a change in mood when the team pulls through a particularly difficult period.

When you're feeling down or dragging, it often helps to lend a hand to others or offer a word of encouragement. They appreciate the help, and you feel needed and appreciated. Know your limitations, and take care of yourself so you can help take care of others. You can only do so much, and there are times when you need to ask for help. Lastly, always, always smile. The world will smile with you, or think you're crazy!

How do I stay positive when my days seem to be forty-eight hours long?

There are two kinds of long days: those that fly by in a blink of an eye and leave you exhilarated but exhausted, and those that tend to drag on forever and leave you deflated by the end. How you spend your time before, during, and after your shift will determine your resilience on those long days. You need to be physically able to handle the emotional and physical stress of your position. For many, this involves attention to exercise, eating well and snacking when necessary, and maintaining good health by getting plenty of sleep and taking vitamin supplements. With such long days devoted to caring for others, you have to find time to care for yourself.

Take advantage of your days off, and treat yourself well. Be sure you use the vacation time that is given to you.

During your shift, you also deserve a moment to remember why you love your job. Stop by the kennel and take a dog for a walk, or pet a cat for a few minutes. With all the known benefits of owning pets and the effect on reducing stress, you would think we would have the most Zen jobs of all! Yet we have to remember to indulge ourselves in these pets we love from time to time.

It helps to remember that this is not a typical nine-to-five job. We are here for the clients and pets when they need us most. Speaking of clients, connecting with a family can be an invigorating pick-me-up during a long day. Helping a client out to the car with a pet or bag of food can enhance the connection, and give you a breath of fresh air at the same time. During a slow day that tends to drag you down, keep your interest up by practicing blood smears or researching an interesting case that you've seen. The pace can become monotonous if you're doing the same task all day long. Try to mix up your duties as much as possible to keep your attention to detail sharp. Finally, those long days often call for good support hose, and a well-stocked kitchen at home for the family!

How can I manage stress
and leave my work at work?

Although those long days can make it seem like we spend all of our time at work, the truth is that work is only part of our lives. We cannot switch off the technician within us as we clock out at the end of our shift, but for the sake of our friends and families, and our psyches, we need to put the day behind us and focus our attention elsewhere as we drive out of the clinic parking lot. A great way to shift gears is to listen to books on CD or music as we make the transition from work to home life.

Even on a day that is not so good, you can get lost in a story or song. You can start focusing on your time at home. Perhaps you begin planning the evening meal or the next activity on your agenda. If you have children, you may start to form questions in your mind to ask about their day. Even if the children or spouse ask you about your day at work, do not let the answer to that question throw you back into the chaos you managed to escape at shift's end. Remember something good or funny to relate, and then let the rest go. Maybe you'll go home to kiss your own pets, and spend quality time with them which can be soothing to your soul.

What about managing stress when you can't leave work? One option is to plan to be the last one in the practice at night, or the first to arrive in the quiet of the morning. Being in the workplace when it's quiet and not stressful can help you see the environment from a new perspective, and help you to find peace even when the chaos starts back up again.

How do I stay inspired when I'm tired, the clients are driving me nuts, and I feel like I'm losing control?

To stay inspired or regain your inspiration, remember why you entered this field to begin with. It is likely you had a desire to help and heal pets, so realize that you accomplish this goal every single day you show up for work. Instead of getting bogged down in the quicksand that can be the daily grind, think of the big picture and realize that you are also helping people by helping pets. These are pet owners who, like you, love their pets very much. You are an important person in their family, as you help their pet through surgery or provide care that helps them to live longer together. Each time a client thanks you for helping to save their pet is a special moment. If you receive cards or letters from clients, create a personal scrapbook that you can turn to during the tough times. You can also find strength in numbers, within your own team of professionals. Participate in team activities, such as parties, sports activities, and events so you can become even closer and support each other on the difficult days. Continuing education can also be inspiring, because you realize that you are offering the highest level of care to your clients and their furry family members. Plus, learning new things can be exciting! The most inspiring moments are usually with the animals, when a cat purrs in response to your touch, or a dog wags his or her tail when he or she sees your friendly face.

Why does burnout happen, and why is there no help for those of us suffering from burnout?

The reasons for burnout are fairly obvious if you consider the struggles of our profession: pets in crisis, outcomes that cannot be medically guaranteed, and families in turmoil. Even when the pet is healthy, there are other factors that lead to professional challenges, including long hours, heavy workloads, and dirty work. The U.S. Department of Labor sums it up by saying of our profession, "Animal lovers get satisfaction in this occupation, but aspects of the work can be unpleasant, physically and emotionally demanding, and sometimes dangerous." Add to that the nearly universal feeling that we are not yet receiving the pay, benefits, respect, and recognition that we deserve, and you have a fine recipe for burnout or compassion fatigue. Most importantly, burnout happens when we do not recognize all of these pressures. We need to respect the serious nature of these challenges and take care of our own physical and mental needs to ensure we have the strength to withstand stress.

There is help available, if you understand where your burnout originates. Internally, you need to address all of these factors. Acknowledge the grief that you feel when trauma or death happens in your practice. Express the frustration that you endure, in a healthy and constructive way, by talking with your coworkers or the practice's management team. Develop a support system outside of your work: family and friends that can help you vent the hurt and refocus on positive aspects of your life. Enjoy activities outside of work, so that you refuel yourself spiritually. Enjoy a hobby that is not work-related, to help you focus on something outside of your day-to-day challenges on the clock. Within the profession, there are professionals who do recognize this serious issue in our profession and are trying to help you. In many conferences now, you will find topics that address grief, compassion fatigue, and burnout. Be sure to attend these lectures. They are just as important as lectures on medical topics.

I have been a RVT for eleven years and want to remain in this field; how do I avoid burnout, and still challenge myself professionally?

As we stay longer in this profession, the chances become greater that we will hit the wall of burnout, and we will look for someplace to turn. Too often, the technician leaves the profession altogether. There is a high level of attrition among veterinary technicians.

There is another way to deal with this situation. One of the best ways to avoid burnout is to challenge yourself professionally. Learn about new techniques and products. Learning is invigorating, and knowing new skills and information reinforces your sense of self-value. When you value your own self, then you will expect to be valued by your employer. If you are not valued, then it is difficult for your work to make you happy.

It may be time to move on, not out of the profession, but on to another practice or type of work within veterinary medicine. You need to recognize that you entered this profession because of your nurturing personality, and as such you probably take on more than you should. Your life is a combination of many things—work, family, your own pets, hobbies, household chores, etc.—and there is a delicate balance that you must assess, and re-prioritize when necessary. Place yourself in the middle, not first so you feel selfish, and not last so there is nothing left of you to give.

How do I make work fun again?

A good sense of humor helps to keep everything in perspective. Yet an enjoyable workplace requires energy on the part of the employees and management. Before you can add the fun back into your daily work, you may have to address those issues that are sapping the enjoyment out of your routine. This may require conversations with your management team or coworkers. Think of your biggest frustrations, and see how they can be reduced or eliminated. Are there work flow issues that are bringing you down, because you cannot create the efficient flow of work that you want? Are there equipment or supply issues that are interfering with the level of patient care you want to provide? Is there squabbling, gossiping, or tension within the team that is a constant source of discouragement? Work cannot be fun if you have a thorn in your side (so to speak) that is causing you discomfort on a daily basis. Once you recognize some of these issues, and help to find solutions, you will feel more lighthearted. Then you can begin to have some real fun again.

Get to know your coworkers on a different level, by spending time away from work. During lunch or break times, talk about things other than work. When you know your coworkers better, it's easier to find ways to make them smile…fun is no fun alone, so try to make someone else laugh every day. Bring in a funny cartoon to post in the employee lounge, grab an image off the Internet of someone's favorite actor or character and tape it on to someone's locker, have mini-celebrations for your colleagues' birthdays or special accomplishments, or schedule a fun activity during a staff meeting or in-house continuing education event. The opportunities are endless.

In order to have fun, you have to feel good about your place of work and the people around you, so the first step is to reach that harmony that allows you to go to the fun place inside yourself.

3

PROMOTING THE PROFESSION

We can obtain many of the things that we as technicians want and deserve—better compensation, more utilization of our skills, recognition of our education or experience, more job opportunities—through promotion of our profession. There are two groups that we want to help understand how far we have come as professionals. One is the veterinary medical team; we need to promote the career of veterinary technology to veterinarians and support staff so that they understand our knowledge and skills, as well as to our fellow technicians so that they can work with us for a better future. The second audience is the general public, especially pet owners. Imagine a time, and perhaps it has even happened now, when a pet owner will only use a practice where credentialed technicians are doing the more advanced tasks. Or when a pet owner insists on a veterinary technician specialist (VTS) in dentistry or anesthesia to be the one caring for the patient during procedures. While VTSs are relatively new, credentialed technicians have been around a long while. There is no reason why the general public should not recognize us for who we are, and how we help their family.

How do we encourage technicians to become more involved in the veterinary community at some level in order to promote themselves and their coworkers?

We all want the same thing, yet some of us have a clearer vision of how to obtain the compensation, recognition, and respect we feel we deserve. Involvement is the key. Like any group with a common goal, technicians must bind together for the common cause. Yet, too many of us are not getting involved within the profession to make a change on a wider scale. The first step is to become a member of your national and state technician association. By joining your voice together with others, we have a better chance of implementing change for the benefit of all. Networking with other technicians at the national and local levels is also important, because you come to realize that the issues go far beyond the walls of your practice. Talk to other technicians whenever you have the opportunity, and share ideas of how to promote the profession. Within your own practice, bring up common issues with your coworkers. If you know of colleagues who are not members of our professional associations, then share information with them that might interest them in becoming involved. Perhaps there is a local or state association meeting nearby, and you can gather up some of your coworkers and share a ride to the event. Share your copies of national technician publications with them, to spark their interest. You can even become a mentor for veterinary technicians before they earn their credentials, by giving presentations at local veterinary technology programs about the importance of being involved in the profession. Be proud of what you do, and promote it whenever the chance arises.

How do I educate the public on the difference between a credentialed technician and an assistant, so that we can be utilized and paid what credentialed technicians deserve?

Most of us are familiar with National Veterinary Technician Week in October every year, when we make a special effort to recognize the technicians on our staff. Many practices also use this week to educate their clientele about the staff in the back. This concept does not only apply to one week out of the year. There are many ways that we can create public awareness of credentialed technicians. How can this in turn create better utilization and higher compensation of credentialed technicians?

Imagine a time when a pet owner comes in to the practice and insists on a credentialed technician drawing the blood sample or administering the vaccination on their pet. Our goal is that veterinarians and state practice acts will insist on credentialed technicians for certain duties. The general public also has a voice that could lead to recognition of our profession. So we need to educate the public. There is widespread ignorance about our profession, and we have the opportunity to change that.

Among our own clientele, we have a captive audience every time they are in our practice. On our walls we can post the Veterinary Technician Oath and other promotional materials from the National Association of Veterinary Technicians in America (NAVTA).

We can introduce our own credentialed technicians with a display of photos, names, and titles. Photos of staff members with their own pets are a great personal touch. With a plaque attached to the frame with the staff member's name and title on it, their credentials will be noticed. Devote a place on your Web site for introducing staff; a short biography can include their educational accomplishments. List the school they attended if appropriate, or the fact that they passed state and/or national board exams to become a credentialed technician. Just as the doctors in your practice should be introduced and recognized by the clientele for their alma mater, education, experience, and credentials, so too should the technicians. Create a brochure or small handout that focuses on the veterinary technology profession, or include this information in your client newsletter. A practice that employs a credentialed technician can use this fact to market their value and expertise to the pet-owning population. When fees are given or questioned, the fact that your staff includes credentialed technicians should be a leading point as well.

RESOURCES
National Association of Veterinary Technicians in America, www.navta.net

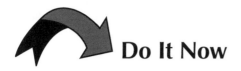 **Do It Now**

Take digital pictures of your employees with their personal pet(s). Designate a place on the lobby wall to display each framed picture, including a nameplate with the employee's name and credentials. Add these same digital pictures to the practice's Web site to introduce employees and their credentials to your clientele.

How do I go about teaching the community about my profession, to gain more people in my field?

As veterinary technicians leave the profession for various reasons, those of us who are left behind are acutely aware that there is a shortage of veterinary technicians entering the workforce. We see staff vacancies in our practices that remain unfilled, and we may work beside unqualified new hires that provide that "warm body" needed for the moment. We may even want to move up or move on in our career, but we need a good technician to fill our old shoes. There are opportunities to teach the general public about veterinary technology as a career choice. The best time to start is when they are young. It is likely that many of us knew we wanted to work with animals from a very young age. You can develop age-appropriate events and materials to teach about veterinary technology. Contact your local elementary, middle, and high schools regarding career days and job fairs. Create or locate fun educational handouts such as coloring books, storybooks, stickers, and brochures to give to students. Arrange with local groups to have tours of your practice. Interested groups could include Boy Scouts, Girl Scouts, 4-H clubs, FFA groups, or classrooms. Give them something to take home as well, so they can share their excitement with their families. This is a good marketing method to reach potential new clients, but it also stimulates young minds to realize the career potential of being a veterinary technician. There are more individualized ways to reach young minds through job co-ops, externships, and volunteer positions within your practice. You will also reach the general public through community events such as pet expos, dog walks, and fairs. Focus your efforts on educating the community about the veterinary technician career.

How do we encourage technicians to promote themselves as professionals (in the way they talk, act, dress, and write) so that they take ownership of their profession?

We refer to veterinary technology as a profession; we must be sure we are portraying ourselves as professionals. This applies whether you are in vet tech school, on duty at your practice, or away from work. Veterinary technician programs are recognizing the importance of graduating well-rounded professionals and are addressing professional development in school. While in the practice, we want recognition from the veterinarians, management team, and support staff.

How often do we take a good look in the mirror to see our reflections? Are we dressing, acting, and communicating like professionals? We are fortunate that we can be professionals without the assistance of a power suit or tie, but appearance is still important. It is difficult to command respect when we have wrinkled scrubs that are stained and covered with fur. It is also impossible to earn the respect of others if we are throwing temper tantrums, pouting to get our way, or appear apathetic and unfeeling.

The management team will almost always address an individual's unprofessional behavior in private, but they can also discuss professionalism as a whole with the entire team. But at some point, we have to take personal responsibility for being a professional. We can demonstrate our professionalism by using appropriate medical terminology in our vocabulary and creating well-written documents without misspellings or grammatical errors. When we are off duty, we are representing our practice and our profession when we wear clothes that contain the practice name or logo, or display our name tag.

At continuing education events, are you wearing casual business attire? While power suits may be reserved for the vendors and salesmen, you should still take pride in how you represent the credentials on your name badge. What can you personally do to encourage technicians to promote themselves as professionals? Lead by example. Professionalism does go both ways. In order to feel like a professional, most of us believe that we must be treated as professionals in terms of pay, utilization, and respect. But we need to keep in mind that this is the same exercise as the chicken and the egg: Which came first, the technician who behaved like a professional, or the technician who was treated like one? If we wait for others, we may deny ourselves the professional recognition we deserve.

How do I get my boss to utilize me to my full potential?

A common recurring theme in the veterinary technology profession is that we do not get utilized to our fullest ability and expertise in daily practice. Technicians may feel like they are viewed as no more than glorified animal handlers. Technician utilization can be further hampered by state practice acts or the lack thereof. State practice acts legally designate which tasks must be performed by a credentialed technician, and which tasks must be performed by a veterinarian. The complaint of underutilization assumes certain things about the veterinarian: that they understand what abilities and knowledge you possess, they understand the practice act as it applies to technicians, and that they are therefore refusing to acknowledge either or both of these facts. These are large assumptions, and they must be addressed to implement a change in your practice.

Start by educating your veterinarians and management team if needed. Remember that unless they attended a veterinary technology program, or passed the technician state and/or national board exams, they have no concept of what your credentials mean to you, to them, and to the practice. Open up a discussion about what can be learned on the job, and what is learned in school or in preparation for the board exam(s), since there are currently states that do not require attendance of an AVMA-recognized veterinary technology program to become credentialed. Acknowledge that veterinary technology school is similar to veterinary school in that graduates may not yet have an advanced level of skill and experience, but they have demonstrated the ability to learn and understand the knowledge behind the skill set they will learn on the floor.

Step up and demonstrate your skills and knowledge to the veterinarians, and have them participate in training of the team. As they teach the technicians, they will learn what their medical staff already knows. It benefits the practice to utilize their technicians as much as possible because it frees up the veterinarians to do what they are trained to do—those tasks that no one else can legally perform. This allows the practice to see more patients. Ultimately, respect from the veterinarians must be earned, and this respect leads to trust. Once the veterinarian trusts you, she is more likely to utilize you fully. Demonstrate that you are a professional, and that you take your credentials seriously. Attend continuing education. During the conference or seminar, network with other veterinarians outside your practice and discuss how utilization of your skills is helping your practice and other veterinarians. Bring back new ideas and information to share with the veterinarians in your practice in a constructive, educational manner. When you strive for excellence, veterinarians are more likely to respect you and the profession.

How do we encourage technicians to embrace and understand the laws that govern the veterinary community?

There are a number of laws that govern veterinary technology, the veterinary community, and the practice of veterinary medicine. These include the state practice acts, which define the roles of veterinarians and veterinary technicians, and the state boards or regulatory agencies in each state that identify the credentialing requirements for veterinary technicians. In addition, there are veterinary medical ethics which outline the type of behavior that is appropriate, and behavior which will not be tolerated by members of the profession. Although the American Veterinary Medical Association (AVMA) has written ethics for the profession at large, it is at the state level that most ethical standards and legal regulations are implemented and enforced. Veterinary technicians must take it upon themselves to learn the applicable laws and ethics of their state of residence. This is not typically difficult to do, with the Internet providing access to state regulatory boards and veterinary medical associations where information can be obtained. The technician must be motivated to go in search of this information. It is difficult for us to obtain respect and recognition if we do not know the laws and ethics that govern our profession. We must realize that there are legal ramifications to the work we do, both for ourselves and our supervising attending veterinarians. We have a role in protecting the medical license of our employer and our own credentials. There are issues surrounding what tasks we can perform, the type of medical records we must keep, and the way we must handle controlled substances, just to name a few. In the practice, these can be topics for continuing education events, staff meetings, or roundtable discussions. There can be a section on an employee bulletin board or in the company newsletter that is devoted to reminders and updates of legal and ethical issues. Without being aware of where we stand in the legal realm of veterinary medicine, we cannot push for changes in the profession or reach the level of importance within the practice that we desire.

RESOURCES
American Association of Veterinary State Boards, http://www.aavsb.org/DLR/DLR.aspx
    (for an index of state veterinary technician regulatory agencies)

AVMA Principles of Veterinary Medical Ethics, www.avma.org/issues/policy/ethics.asp
Directory to links of state associations, www.avma.org/statevma/default.asp
Law and Ethics of the Veterinary Profession, by James F. Wilson, DVM, JD (Priority Press Ltd. 1993)

How can we keep credentialed technicians from leaving the profession?

We know of a technician that has been at the same practice for over thirty years, yet she is the only one from her class still employed in the profession. When we lose good technicians, our entire profession suffers, as do the clients and pets. In order to understand how to retain credentialed technicians in the profession, we have to understand that there are a variety of reasons they leave.

Some leave due to what they see as the financial limitations of our career. Yet, in actuality, if financial compensation is the only reason they left, then there are probably options they did not explore. Did they investigate the expansion of their own credentials, skills, and knowledge to obtain higher pay? Did they consider trying to move up in their practice via a step into management? (Of course, managing does not suit everyone.) Did they explore career changes into other avenues of veterinary medicine that perhaps pay more than companion animal practice? Were they willing to relocate to find a better paying opportunity? (However, often the veterinary technician in the family is the second, lower-income earner in the household, so the family cannot move in search of a career change in veterinary medicine.)

If burnout or compassion fatigue has led them to exit the profession, did they reach outward or inward for help in coping with their emotional exhaustion? Did they consider changing employers to find a better fit for them psychologically, such as a practice with less stress or better staff scheduling?

A certain level of attrition in our profession is to be expected when you consider that the majority of veterinary technicians are women, and many of them have desires to raise families while they are active in the profession. Whether the technician in question is a male or a female, this is a major factor to be considered. How family-friendly was their practice at the time? Were they given sufficient time off for the birth or adoption of the child and for medical issues that may have arisen during pregnancy? Could their practice support a change in schedule if requested or required once the child joined the family? Basically, was it possible for the employee to be a parent and an employed technician at the same time?

People leave the profession for various reasons, and those of us who remain in the profession must realize that a person's individual situation affects the attrition rate just as much as factors such as perceived low pay or inadequate recognition.

Why are credentialed veterinary technicians not compensated for their hard work?

Sometimes the issues involve recognition, utilization, and public aware-ness. But this question also goes hand-in-hand with another question, "How do I help all team members feel just as important as the doctors when it comes to the bottom line?" If you work in a practice where you are utilized to your fullest potential by a wonderful group of doctors who respect you and encourage your professional growth, then your compensation is most affected by the profitability of the practice.

Veterinary practices are businesses, and as such they function within certain budget limitations. Payroll for staff is nearly half of the basic budget of a veterinary practice, and a good leadership team would like to pay you even more per hour. How can you help them do this? By contributing to the growth of this budget. Too often technicians assume the only thing standing in the way of higher pay is the person writing the check; but it is the dollar figure in the bank, the actual cash flow of the business, that limits that number on your paycheck. Fifty percent of a larger sum means more money for each person on the team. Technicians can take at least part of the responsibility for the financial stability of the business. This is because everything you do affects this bottom line. Every catheter you have to replace because you forgot to put an e-collar on a patient, every expired bottle of reconstituted medica-tion that you have to discard because you mixed a new one without looking first, every client that you alienate because you're having a bad day, costs the practice money. Yet there are just as many ways that you can contribute to the financial well-being of the business. You can conserve white goods or dispos-able supplies, you can keep tight control of inventory, and you can provide excellent service to every client, every time, to help the practice have more money in the bank. And they will likely share the profits with you and your colleagues! We come full circle to that question raised earlier about asking for a well-deserved raise: When you've helped contribute to the profitability of the practice, be sure to ask for your share! Last, we were asked, "When are credentialed veterinary technicians going to get the respect and compensation they deserve?" This question is yours to answer.

4

CLIENT SERVICE

It is easy to think we are in the business of taking care of animals. That is true, to a point. We are mainly in the business of taking care of people, who then allow us to care for their pets. Without their owners' permission, we would not be trusted to provide the care that is needed by those animals. Therefore, the way we treat the clients will determine if we have access to the animals. It is also true that pets cannot tell their owners about their experience in "the back." They cannot say, "The technicians treated me gently and gave me the care that healed me," or, "The assistants petted me all the time and took me out for walks whenever I needed to go," or, "Those sweet front-office people smile every time they walk past my cage and talk nice to me!" Indeed, the only reality the pet owners experience is how they are treated, not their pets. How do we know this is true even in extreme situations? You can recover a pet from a devastating illness or injury and provide life-saving care that brings the animal back to health. Yet, if you mistreat the client, she will not return to your practice. On the other hand, you can lose a pet to death despite your best efforts, or even occasional misjudgments, and yet, if you treat that client well, he will return with his next pet or will recommend friends and family. The only gauge clients have to measure our medical care is through our client care. So we must be attentive to the needs of our pet-owning population.

How do I triage a patient in front of the client without worrying the pet's family?

Two types of triage happen routinely in the lobby of a veterinary practice: the medical triage of the pet, and the emotional triage of the pet owner or family. Even when the patient is visibly stable upon arrival, the veterinary team should treat the situation as if it were an emergency if that is how the family is feeling. This does not mean panic should ensue, but instead an orderly and concerned process that assesses the patient's condition while respecting the emotions of the client. If the pet arrives in visible distress—seizing, bleeding, gasping for breath, etc.—the patient should be taken to the back while a front office or client service team member tends to the family. When the patient appears stable, the triage may occur in the lobby to determine if the pet can wait with the family to see the doctor, or needs to go back to be monitored by the medical staff. During the initial phone call, or when they enter the practice, the pet owners should be notified of this triage process and the possibility that they may need to be separated from their pet, if necessary.

In the lobby, the technician should approach the family and introduce herself to both the people and the pet. Explain in layman's terms exactly what you will be doing with their pet, and what you are looking for as you go along. While obtaining a basic history of the immediate problem during conversation with the clients, the technician can assess the basic status of the pet. It is best to avoid having to count respiratory or heart rates during this initial assessment, because it is difficult to count accurately while giving the clients your attention as well. Once completed, inform the clients of the assessment without alarming them or instilling false hope. Instead of saying, "Fluffy looks fine," tell the clients, "Fluffy appears to be stable at the moment, so she can wait with you for the doctor; however, if Fluffy's condition changes, notify the front desk immediately and we'll be back." Instead of saying, "I need to take Fluffy to the back right away!" in a panic, tell the client, "I believe Fluffy needs immediate monitoring in our treatment area, but we'll have an update for you in just a few moments." Maintain an even composure without appearing apathetic. You always want to express concern and sympathy for what the family is going through, while tending to your animal patient.

How should I treat
time-consuming clients?

There is no doubt that our days can be plagued with time-consuming clients. The first thing you need to do is resist your initial reaction to groan, and realize that for some people this is the highlight of their day. You may be the one person who truly understands how important that pet is to them. Yet you also have other clients and patients who need your attention. The trick is to give them the impression that you have all the time in the world, while prioritizing the four other things you must immediately attend to behind the scenes. It will help if you are organized and have backup plans. Develop casual scripts that you can use to transition from one part of the visit to the next. After your initial portion of the visit, announce that you'll get the doctor now and prop open the door to leave. If they begin to ramble about the pet's symptoms, politely tell them that you know the doctor will want to hear the details (as long as it's not your job to obtain the complete history from the client). Or hand them an informational brochure that pertains to their visit or a new promotion at the practice, to distract their attention and move forward with your exit.

When the visit is complete, escort them to the front desk to check out as you go over instructions or products you are sending home. If they deviate from the conversation about the pet, bring them back on track by asking if they have any last questions. Introduce them to the person who will be checking them out to make the transition smooth and seamless. It helps if you have everything gathered and ready for each step of the appointment. Then you will not have to disengage over and over again from the conversation.

If you have a few clients who you know require extra time of the staff to be provided excellent client service, make a note on their record. This way a short amount of time can be added to their appointment slot or you can tag-team with a colleague to have them put the next appointment in while you finish chatting at the front desk. For a client who seems to think of one question, then another, then another, casually ask him to come next time with a list of questions that you can review while the doctor is examining their pet. In this way you can gather up educational materials or obtain answers to their questions while the appointment is proceeding. You'll also be able to keep them focused on the questions they really want answered during their visit.

How should I respond when a person calls to "price shop" a common service?

If the caller has never visited your practice, they are not merely a price shopper but a potential new client. If they are an existing client, their call gives you the opportunity to strengthen your relationship with that family. The actual price of the item being requested is one of the last, and least important, facts that you will relay to the caller.

First, ask questions, because people respond to attention. The more you communicate with the caller, the better you can determine their needs and provide help. Find out the caller's name, their pet's name, species, and age. Then find a way to educate them on the product or service they are requesting. For prescription diets or products, your veterinarian will need to examine the pet to establish the veterinarian-client-patient relationship. Describe this examination process, and relate it to the pet's species and age. Use this opportunity to educate them about your wellness or geriatric program, for example, before you give a price.

This opportunity to educate the client is particularly important when discussing prices for surgical services. You want to be sure that they are comparing apples to apples between practices, so you need to describe all that is involved in the procedure at your practice. List the appropriate pre-operative lab test, the intravenous catheter and fluid support, the pulse oximeter monitoring equipment, the standard pain control, etc. and why all of this is important to their pet. If they respond that they have received lower prices from other practices, politely ask them if those clinics provide the extra items that you have mentioned. If there is adequate lead time before the prospective appointment, offer to send them brochures or additional educational materials about your practice and the surgery they are requesting. These materials can explain the surgery in detail, so they understand what is involved in the cost and the best care of their pet. Offer to have them stop by the practice, tour the facility, and meet members of the staff. Make them feel welcome from the moment you answer the phone. You will find that most callers are not as interested in the price as they are interested in finding the place that will best take care of them and their pet. They will pay more for services if they feel an emotional value for the services you provide.

How do I deal with very difficult clients, the ones who truly upset the staff, and cause chaos and instability in the practice? Do I "fire" them?

The decision to "fire" a client needs to come from the owner of the practice, in consultation with the management team, but every employee has the right and responsibility to report incidents involving clients to a member of management so that a decision can be reached. Incidents can include those that cause disruption to work flow, result in emotional trauma to employees, or create dangerous situations for the staff or other clients in the facility.

Your practice needs to have a protocol in place for how to handle these incidents. The protocol should answer the following questions. How is the event documented? Who is it reported to? Are notes entered into the medical record of the client or patient? When should local police authorities be called? Include any other pertinent considerations. There is no doubt that clients can and do abuse veterinary staff members verbally, emotionally, and sometimes physically. Your practice has an obligation to provide a safe workplace, free from abuse and harassment.

Your practice owner needs to take all related factors into consideration when determining whether or not to terminate a client's relationship with the practice. This includes the nature of the incident (did the client yell and curse, or threaten physical harm?), the existing relationship with the client (is this his first visit, or has he been a client for years?), the economical impact on the practice (has he spent very little money at the practice, or thousands of dollars with multiple pets over the years?), how often the client is difficult (was it a first offense, or is this client continually abusive?), the reaction of the staff involved (did the staff member ignite the situation by becoming defensive or yelling back?), and the condition of the patient.

According to the *AVMA Principles of Veterinary Medical Ethics*, a veterinarian cannot terminate the relationship if the patient is experiencing an ongoing medical or surgical condition. She may refer the patient and client to another veterinarian, but the veterinarian is obligated to provide care as needed during this transition. The practice should also protect itself by sending the client a formal letter of termination. Even though the decision to "fire" a client is not as simple as staff members would like to believe, there should be open communication between the staff and the practice leadership regarding any concerns with client behavior.

RESOURCES

AVMA Principles of Veterinary Medical Ethics, www.avma.org/issues/policy/ethics.asp

Law and Ethics of the Veterinary Profession, by James F. Wilson, DVM, JD (Priority Press, Ltd. 1993)

Legal Consents for Veterinary Practices, by James F. Wilson, DVM, JD (Priority Press, Ltd. 2006)

What is the best way for me to handle an angry or upset client on the telephone?

Sometimes your body language can help you to handle an angry client in person at the front desk or in an examination room. However, on the telephone, you only have your words and tone of voice to help you through the situation. There are also times when clients find it easier to be angry and belligerent through the telephone wire rather than in front of your face. This can create some very uncomfortable if not impossible situations for the team members who handle these calls. At the same time, you want to retain or gain these callers for your clientele.

The most important thing to remember is to let the client talk! Often the mere act of venting frustration will help the client to calm down, and you may end up with an apology at the end of his tirade. This is perhaps difficult to do if you are in the middle of a busy day and feel your time is limited. However, this is no time to rush, and it may take teamwork to free up a member of the staff to be the attentive ear that this upset client needs. When he has finished his ranting, repeat his main concerns back to him to demonstrate that you have heard and understood the complaint. Then ask him, in a calm yet attentive voice, how you can help to rectify the situation. He needs to know that you are listening and focused. Be careful not to apologize on behalf of the practice, as this could be viewed as an admission of guilt. Unless you have completed a thorough investigation of this client's complaint, you have no way of knowing who is at fault, if, in fact, anyone is. Acknowledge the client's feelings. You could say something like, "I can tell that you're frustrated; what would you like me to do to help?" or, "It is unfortunate that you feel that way; what can we do for you at this point?" or, "I understand how upset you are about (pet's name) illness; let me see what I/we can do for you." Above all, remain calm, and never become emotional. Do not participate in a shouting match, or battle of wits. The client might not "always be right," but he does need to feel validated and understood.

RESOURCES
Enhancing Your Telephone Skills (CD-ROM), by Mark Opperman, CVPM (Lifelearn 1999)
The Veterinary Receptionist's Handbook, Second Edition, by M. T. McClister, DVM; and Amy Midgley (Veterinary Medicine Publishing Group 2000)

How do I deal with clients who have found misinformation on the Internet?

The best information for your clients to have is the information that your practice can provide. So your first defense against misinformation are the brochures, handouts, and resources that you can provide your clients who want to learn more about the care of their pets. Be sure to give them the names or business cards of your technicians, so they have someone to call when they have a question. When clients arrive or call with misinformation gathered on the Internet, you need to handle the situation in a respectful way. Assure them that you are glad they are looking for more information, and applaud them for wanting to expand their knowledge of caring for their pet. Yet gently inform them that there is no validation process for the information that is typed into a Web page or linked to a Web site, so they need to be careful and vigilant, even slightly skeptical, of the information they read.

These clients obviously use the Internet to gather details, so point them to Web sites that your practice can recommend. Make them familiar with the names and acronyms of organizations that provide good information, such as the American Veterinary Medical Association (AVMA), their state veterinary medical association (VMA), and others. If the client insists on relying on information he found on the Web, politely ask him to bring in the article or give you the link so your staff can check out the material. Then you can dissect the information and point out what may be valid, and what is likely not valid, at least for his pet's specific condition, for example. If a client does not appreciate your redirection, he may feel that your opinion is tainted by the fact that you stand to profit from medications, products, or lab tests purchased or performed at your practice. The client needs to trust your motives, so be careful not to sound like a salesman, and focus solely on the health of his pet. If there are third-party, neutral sources that can corroborate your treatment plan or recommendations—such as reputable Web sites, brochures, or even lectures by experts in the industry—share these with your clients so they can see that your practice's medical opinion comes from valid sources. Your clients are reaching for answers and solutions, particularly if their pet is ill, so validate their feelings and answer any questions they may have about their pet's illness or treatment. If their questions go unanswered by your practice, they will search elsewhere for the comfort they seek. Turn these conversations into great starting points for educating your clients, and help them to become better pet owners.

What resource can my practice recommend to clients for finding medical information?

When clients need information, they should first turn to you and your veterinary practice. Yet, clients often want to validate the information you have shared, or learn more than they may think you can provide. Referring your clients to an outside source can be a way to help them learn more on their own time and at their own speed and comfort level. There are many recommended Internet sites where pet owners can find good information about caring for their pets listed in the resources below. You must be careful, however, if your practice is recommending an outside source, or even handing out brochures or information to your clients, that the staff knows the information contained in this material. You do not want the client knowing more than your staff on any given topic. Be certain that the veterinarians agree with everything stated in the literature if it is obtained from an outside source. You certainly do not want to be in the position of explaining the discrepancy later to a questioning client. If there is no literature that accurately reflects your practice's medical opinion on a topic, then it needs to be created by your veterinarians. Involve the entire team in the review of this material. They may have a perspective to share that could be overlooked. For example, a technician may realize that more home care instructions need to be added, or the receptionist may notice that the tone of the writing is not as user friendly as your clients would prefer. The team is more likely to be invested in the material given out to clients if they help to create it. When everyone receives the same education, the pets benefit the most.

RESOURCES
AAHA Pet Health Brochures (available on many different topics)
American Animal Hospital Association, www.aahanet.org
American Veterinary Medical Association, www.avma.org
Companion Animal Parasite Council, www.capcvet.org
Directory of links to state veterinary medical associations, www.avma.org/statevma/
    default.asp
PetCare Television Network, www.petcaretv.com
PetPlace.com, www.petplace.com

VeterinaryPartner, www.veterinarypartner.com
VetStreet's Pet Portals, www.petportals.com

How can I occupy children in the exam room?

Sometimes your biggest challenges are the little members of the family that do not have fur! Many families who own pets also have children, so it is important to plan ahead for the kids who will visit your practice. It is important to realize that children can be an important part of caring for a family pet. It is in the pet's best interest to use this opportunity to educate the youngsters. Teach them what signs they can notice that could indicate their pet is sick: food left in the bowl, a pet that is not wanting to play or yelps when touched, or discharge from different places on the body, especially the face. With busy parents trying to keep up with the entire family, it is often the children that will first notice details about the pet's behavior or appearance. If they are old enough to be interested in the examination process, involve them by letting them listen through your stethoscope, or peer into the ears with an otoscope. Of course, keep the children safe. Always provide adequate restraint of their pet. Ask the children questions about the history of the pet and the pet's symptoms, just as you would ask the adults in the family. If you have brochures, especially with pictures (not ones that are too graphic), share them with the kids.

Some children are too young, or just uninterested in participating in the visit. Have a wide variety of activities to keep them occupied. If your practice has a play area in the lobby stocked with toys and books, you can offer for them to bring along their plaything to the examination room. In the exam room, you can provide quiet activities such as crayons, coloring books, puzzles, and stickers to keep little hands and minds busy. Remember to keep safety in mind for your non-furry friends as well, so watch the age requirements on toys and keep all the shared toys and play areas sanitized between visitors. Families who feel their children are welcome at your practice will be more likely to continue the relationship.

CLIENT RESOURCES
Coloring Book and Crayons for Kids (AAHA Press 2000)
Doggie Manners: Dog Bite Safety Activity Sheet (AAHA Press 2008)
Super Hamster in a Visit to the Animal Hospital (AAHA Press 2001)

Web Sites
www.4imprint.com
www.apromotionaloutlet.com
www.branders.com
www.IASpromotes.com
www.motivators.com
www.printablepromotions.com

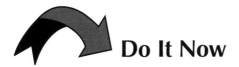 **Do It Now**

Purchase a supply of activities to keep younger clients busy so that work can proceed on their pet: coloring books, washable crayons, stickers, puzzles, books, and age-appropriate, quiet toys.

What is the best way to console a grieving client over the loss of his pet?

There may be no best way to console a client, because every pet owner grieves his pet in a different way. There are five recognized stages of grieving: denial, anger, bargaining, depression or grief, and acceptance or resolution. You will encounter clients who are working through any or many of these stages at any given time, and perhaps you will witness several stages with a single client. Therefore, it can be very difficult to provide the type of support that we need to give to our clients. Keep in mind that it is likely that nothing you do will truly help them at that moment, but they may reflect on your assistance later and be grateful.

You learn how to comfort clients much the same way you learn client service in general—by trying to read the person's body language and respond accordingly. You also need to be comfortable with the type of comforting you are providing. Soothing words that validate the clients' loss and recognize their grief may be right up your alley. Sometimes saying nothing is more appropriate. Some technicians feel a comforting touch on the back or a heartfelt hug is best, and they are comfortable providing that; but if you are not a hugger, do not attempt it. The clients will sense your discomfort, and then you have defeated the purpose. Often just your presence in the room or next to clients is comforting, and being there to listen if they want to talk about their feelings or past memories of their pet.

Realize that this loss is significant for the pet owner, and he will remember these moments of grief. Do not do or say anything that is not appropriate and respectful. Know the pet's name and gender so you can refer to the situation personally, and do not comment on the pet's personality unless you truly knew the animal. If you did know the pet well, you can relay a nice memory of your experience with that animal. This might encourage the client to open up and share stories of memorable times with his pet. Also remain aware of how you handle the deceased pet. Handle the pet's remains as gently as if the pet was still alive. If you are removing the body from the examination room, remember that this may be the last visual memory the client has of a beloved pet. In general, quiet respect and sincere efforts are appreciated the most by grieving clients.

What resources can I recommend for grieving clients?

The veterinary practice staff should be as supportive as possible for clients who are grieving. It is also important to provide these clients with other resources to explore their feelings and deal with their grief process. Your practice can create a sympathy packet to give to clients during this time. In this packet you can include information about local resources such as grief support groups or grief counselors. Your practice can establish a pet loss support group to help clients meet with others who are experiencing the same loss. Your practice's Web site can provide helpful links or a place to memorialize pets. On a wider level, you can provide information on organizations such as the Association of Pet Loss and Bereavement. There are grief hotlines which are established by some veterinary schools and teaching hospitals.

Your practice can provide brochures or recommend books on the topic of grief or helping children cope with the loss of a pet. Your relationship with that family extends beyond the life of that one pet, and providing resources is a way of respecting that relationship.

RESOURCES
The Argus Institute at Colorado State University, www.argusinstitute.colostate.edu/grief.htm
The Association for Pet Loss and Bereavement, www.aplb.org
Coping with the Loss of Your Pet, by Kathleen Ayl, PhD (Grief Associates 2007)
A Final Act of Caring, by Mary and Herb Montgomery (Montgomery Press 1993)
Forever in My Heart, by Mary and Herb Montgomery (Montgomery Press 2000)
Good-bye My Friend, by Mary and Herb Montgomery (Montgomery Press 1991)
The Loss of Your Pet (brochure, AAHA Press 2003)
Paws 2 Heaven state directory of resources, www.paws2heaven.com/Support_directory.htm
The Pet Loss Grief Support Web site, www.petloss.com
PetSupport.net, www.petsupport.net
The Practical Guide to Client Grief, by Laurel Lagoni, MS (AAHA Press 1997)
A Snowflake in My Hand, by Samantha Mooney (Delta 1995)
A Special Place for Charlee, by Debby Morehead (Partners in Publishing, LLC 1996)
University of California Davis (extensive resource list and links), www.vetmed.ucdavis.edu/ccab/petloss.html
When Your Pet Dies, by Alan D. Wolfelt, PhD (Companion Press 2004)

When someone's pet is euthanized, I sometimes feel so sad that I end up crying myself. I really want to be there for the owners, but the sadness overwhelms me. How can I be sympathetic and still hold it together?

It is a mistake to think that you cannot cry when a pet dies, whether it is from euthanasia or natural causes. Being affected by the sadness does not mean that you cannot be sympathetic to your clients. In fact, those clients will appreciate and remember that you were empathetic during their loss.

You may have met this animal when it was young, coming in for the first time as a kitten or puppy full of fun and mischief. Perhaps you watched this pet grow up and helped keep it healthy under the watchful eye of its family. If you nursed this pet during an injury or illness, then you cared for the animal during a time of profound need, when the family could not be by their pet's side. Even if you have never met a pet before it is brought in for humane euthanasia, you can quickly recognize the grief of the family, and know how special this pet must have been during its healthy years. We are in this profession because of our profound love of animals, and it is natural for us to be affected when a pet becomes injured, ill, or dies. Whatever history you may have with this pet is part of your experience of loving animals. Those memories will remain with you forever.

Suppressing your grief will not help the family in your care, nor will it help you to survive the emotions that come along with your job title. If you feel that your emotions are so overwhelming that you cannot provide support for the family, then perhaps you need to take a private moment. But generally speaking, shedding tears in front of the family only proves to them that you care, that you share their sorrow, and that you are in the right line of work.

CHAPTER RESOURCES
Client Satisfaction Pays, by Carin A. Smith, DVM (AAHA Press 1998, 2009)
Connecting with Clients, by Laurel Lagoni, MS; and Dana Durrance, MA (AAHA Press 1998)
Educating Your Clients from A to Z, by Nan Boss, DVM (AAHA Press 1999)
Essentials of Client Service (CD-ROM), by Sheila Grosdidier (Lifelearn 1998)

First Impressions That Last (DVD and Workbook), by Cecelia J. Soares, DVM, MS, MA (AAHA Press 1999)

One Client at a Time (DVD and Workbook), by Cecelia J. Soares, DVM, MS, MA (AAHA Press 1999)

Skills for Communicating with Patients, by Jonathan Silverman, FRCGP; Suzanne Kurtz, PhD; and Juliet Draper, FRCGP, MD (Radcliffe Publishing 2005)

5

STAFF TRAINING

Creating good teams is hard work. As if the recruiting and hiring process was not difficult enough, we must then provide adequate staff training to mold and shape the type of team members we need and desire. New graduates of veterinary technology programs have a foundation of knowledge, but they need our mentoring to realize their full potential. Someone with years of experience at another practice comes in with lots of skills, but still needs to be taught how we do things *here*. Sometimes they have to be untrained in their old ways before they can be trained in new ways. This can be frustrating for everyone involved.

Once we have our team just where we want it, there is *still* training to do. Veterinary medicine is constantly evolving and expanding. There are new medications, new treatments, advanced equipment, and increased knowledge that must constantly be incorporated into any progressive practice that aims to provide quality pet healthcare. So the existing team must continue to be trained in new developments, and the learning must never cease.

How do I make time to train new staff while still completing my responsibilities?

This question itself is an exercise in futility. You cannot complete your full responsibilities while training new staff members. The mentor assigned to train a new hire needs to be given time to do the training without being fully responsible for her usual tasks. She needs scheduled time off of the floor to review learning materials and discuss protocols. There needs to be some time scheduled for light duty, where she can demonstrate tasks and procedures on actual events happening in the practice, allowing extra time to slow down and teach the task. This may require scheduling extra staff on these days or during these periods. There is nothing more frustrating for both the trainer and the trainee than being in the middle of a busy day and trying to teach or learn on the fly!

However, there are times when learning needs to happen during a hectic event. When a patient's life is at stake, there is no time to slow down and teach. Instead, the new hire should keep a small notebook and pen with her at all times to jot down notes and questions during the event. Then, after the crisis is over, she can step aside with her mentor and ask questions about what she observed. This exchange of information should happen as soon after the event as possible, to enhance the retention of learning.

Keep in mind that a new hire should not necessarily be trained by only one person. Team members have different areas of expertise or knowledge, and the new staff person should rotate through trainers to benefit from the entire team's input.

There are also good ways to teach without involving team members who are busy on the floor. There are computer and Internet training sources available, plus you can create your own training materials. The team can identify each step of a process, then take digital pictures and write the text to create a how-to guide. These guides can be kept on the computer or printed and kept in binders for quick reference in appropriate locations. Use various trainers and methods, and remember to set aside appropriate time for effective training to take place.

RESOURCES

Animal Care Technologies online staff training, www.4act.com

Job Descriptions and Training Schedules for the Veterinary Team, by James F. Wilson, DVM, JD; and Karen Gendron, DVM (Priority Press, Ltd. 2005)

The Veterinary Receptionist's Training Manual, by James F. Wilson, DVM, JD; and Carol McConnell, DVM (Priority Press, Ltd. 1995)

How do I train our technicians to do cystocentesis, urinary catheter placements, IV catheter placements, and central line placements without using live animals?

Although video learning, demonstration, and observation can be utilized, it is difficult to teach procedures that seem to require live animals. It is also difficult to evaluate the skill level of an existing team member or new hire. The gold standard may be live animals for learning some procedures, and practices have found ways to provide these subjects through local humane associations or animal shelters. At some level, teaching must occur on our patients, under the close supervision of experienced technicians and veterinarians. However, there are other creative ways to imitate the experience of treating a live animal in the clinic setting. Using an empty paper towel roll, surgical drain, vet wrap, and saline with dye added, you can create "dummy legs" to practice placing intravenous catheters and accessing veins for venipuncture or administering medications. Stuffed animals provide very tame subjects to practice restraint and bandaging. Yet, these stuffed patients can also be modified in some creative ways to provide a practice area for entubation, enema application, and intravenous catheter placement using red rubber tubes as veins. For more advanced procedures, there are models that look stuffed on the outside, but are quite complex with internal modifications. Although some of these models are expensive, you may be able to form an alliance with other local practices or associations so that you can share these advanced learning tools. It is likely that nothing will replace the real thing, but there are ways to demonstrate and practice techniques that can later be applied to our patients in need.

RESOURCES
Rescue Critters Animal Training "Mannikins," www.rescuecritters.com

How do I get employees to follow hospital protocol? What is the best way to get staff to buy into new procedures and protocols?

One question answers the other: Employees will follow hospital protocol if they buy into the procedures and protocols in the practice. You obtain staff buy-in when you involve them in developing and implementing the procedures and protocols. They will perform a job better when they feel ownership than when they feel the job is forced upon them. It's the difference between being told what to do, and being asked what you feel is the best way to accomplish the same objective.

If you are able to provide your input and opinion, and hear the opinions of others, then you are more likely to reach a consensus that everyone agrees to carry out. This takes time, and it takes a structured approach. The management team can present an idea as a draft for review by the team. It is helpful to explain why this particular protocol was developed, and the necessary goals or outcomes. Solicit the team's questions and concerns during a staff or section meeting. When this meeting is over and consensus is reached, post the minutes of the meeting and require every team member to read and sign the document, even if they were present at the meeting. This reinforces compliance and ensures that everyone receives the same information.

Once the final protocol has been revised and written, the team needs to be trained completely in the new process. Depending on the nature of the task, handouts, posted information, or reference sheets can be provided. A demonstration may also be necessary. The team leaders, doctors, and senior staff members should lead by example and provide gentle verbal reminders when necessary. Be sure to add this new protocol to existing training programs and standard operating procedures' notebooks and reference materials. Do not assume that one training session is always enough. Repeat the training in a few weeks, for example. Expect accountability from the team. You can evaluate their level of understanding and competency by giving them a short quiz or verbal test, or by asking them to demonstrate the skill for a grade.

RESOURCES
How We Do Things Here: Developing and Teaching Office-Wide Protocols, by Nan Boss, DVM (AAHA Press 2009)

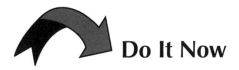 **Do It Now**

Develop a consistent protocol for all new
or changed protocols. Create a form
that documents each step of the process:
Inform and Explain, Discuss and Revise,
Post and Sign, Train and Retrain, Test;
Add to SOPs and Training Program.
Each form should have the protocol title at
the top and the dates when each step was
completed to ensure consistency
through the team.

How do I locate
continuing education opportunities?

A portion of ongoing training will come from outside continuing education opportunities. This is an important way to enhance knowledge and skills and bring new concepts back into the practice for consideration. Large national conferences provide many days of lectures, wet labs, and presentations. Information on these events is usually easy to locate because they advertise extensively in journals and through direct mail. There are other great educational events that may be closer to home and more affordable for you and your practice. There are regional events that bring together many states in the same part of the country, so the travel distance is not as far. Many local organizations sponsor continuing education seminars that may only require a day or an evening of your time. You can learn about many events through your local and state veterinary associations; national, state, and local technician associations; local veterinary technology schools or veterinary schools; technician specialty academies; veterinary industry associations and publications; and vendors or sales representatives.

RESOURCES
Academy of Internal Medicine for Veterinary Technicians, www.aimvt.com
Academy of Veterinary Behavior Technicians, www.avbt.org
Academy of Veterinary Dental Technicians, www.avdt.us
Academy of Veterinary Emergency and Critical Care Technicians, www.avecct.org
American Veterinary Medical Association, www.avma.org
Academy of Veterinary Technician Anesthetists, www.avta-vts.org
Directory of links to state veterinary medical associations, www.avma.org/statevma/
    default.asp
National Association of Veterinary Technicians in America, www.navta.net
NAVTA Journal, www.navta.net
Veterinary Communities—Veterinary Information Network, www.vin.com
Veterinary Practice News, www.veterinarypracticenews.com
Veterinary Support Personnel Network, www.vspn.org
Veterinary Technicians and Assistants Resource Center, www.vtarc.com
Veterinary Technician Journal, www.vettechjournal.com
VetMedTeam, www.vetmedteam.com

What is the best way to approach management concerning continuing education for technicians?

Most practice owners and management teams recognize the importance of continuing education and encourage their technicians to continue learning. However, they may have varying abilities to provide the necessary support, namely, the time away from work and financial assistance to attend. Both of these represent a potential financial loss or expense on the part of the practice, as they may be required to pay someone additional hours, wages, or overtime to cover your shift(s), or provide an allowance for your educational endeavors. In the mind of a businessperson such as your practice owner, they want to see a return on their investment. This is true for any expenditure in the practice, including your continued learning.

If you want or need to request additional financial assistance, then you will certainly need to justify your request. You can start by reviewing the specific knowledge and skills that you and the rest of the team have been able to apply from past continuing education experiences. It is even better if you can take it one step further and calculate the profits or revenue made by the implementation of these new ideas in the past. Even if you are allotted a certain amount of continuing education allowance each year, make this topic a part of your annual or scheduled performance evaluation. Discuss the continuing education you have attended during the evaluation period, and demonstrate how you have applied your additional skills or knowledge.

Confirm the allowance amount for the upcoming period. This is an appropriate time to address any requests for additional money as well. If you know there is an event that would benefit you and the practice to attend, and you will need additional funds to go, do your homework first. Calculate how much the continuing education event will cost in total, including travel (gas or airfare), hotel, registration, additional wet labs or events, food, etc. Never expect the practice to give you the total amount necessary, but do demonstrate that you are willing to invest in your own education. If you have to fund the remaining amount, they will know you are committed to ongoing learning. Aside from the financial return on the investment, it is important to note to your practice manager or owner that continuing education has less tangible benefits. An educated staff provides higher-quality care to patients and clients. Learning can invigorate the team and help them to maintain a more fulfilling and satisfying career. Team members who are encouraged about their future tend to work harder, be more devoted to their profession and practice, and stay longer in their position or at their practice.

How do I convince the practice to implement changes or integrate information after I have attended a continuing education event?

Even if your practice supports your attendance at continuing education events, it does not necessarily mean that new ideas or skills will be implemented upon your return. It can be frustrating to return excited and motivated from a continuing education opportunity, only for your practice leadership to turn a deaf ear to your suggestions. Before you approach the management team, you need to assess whether these new skills or ideas fit the practice's goals or mission. Typically, a mission is general or broad enough that it has space for new ideas, if you know how to present them. For example, if your practice mission, motto, or tagline is "to provide quality medical care," then it can be argued that the leadership team would want to advance the skills of their technician staff. This is your starting point when you present your ideas. Show the leadership team how the new procedures, equipment, medication, or treatment options that you learned about can have a direct impact on improving the medical care provided by the practice. Feel free to quote the practice's mission during this presentation. Map out the implementation of this idea in a written document. An outline format is sufficient and will provide the management team enough detail so that they can decide whether to pursue the idea further.

It is one thing to come back and say, "Wow, I saw this great new piece of machinery that can monitor patients better than the junky old pulse ox that we have"; it is entirely another thing to come back and present a document that says: "Our mission is to provide quality medical care to our patients. There are new advances in monitoring equipment that can help us reach this goal." Then provide information on the manufacturer, distributer, cost (including installation, service, supplies, and quality control), and features. Outline how the staff can be adequately trained on this new equipment. Will it require an in-house demonstration for the entire staff all at one time, or can multiple training sessions be worked into the staff schedule? Explain how this new equipment will assist the team, benefit the patients, and improve the profitability of the practice. The same concept applies to a new procedure or skill that is learned at a continuing education event. Outline what the procedure is and why implementing it in the practice would improve patient care. Go through the same steps of discussing necessary supplies, training objectives, and financial benefits. The management team needs information to make a decision on implementing new ideas, and you are the best one to give them this information when you return from a fantastic learning event.

How can I find time to read and keep up with all of the veterinary publications that will keep me up-to-date with the veterinary profession?

We all have more work than hours given in a day. We have our shift in the practice, then our family and friends, household chores and children's activities, and even our own pets to care for. Where do you find time to take a break, much less keep up with your profession or your special interest in veterinary medicine?

First, you have to make it a priority, at least somewhere near the upper portion of your list of things to do. If you do not mentally prioritize the pursuit of continuing education, it will not happen. And you could get left behind in this industry that is constantly evolving and adapting. Examine your daily or weekly schedule and see where you might be able to maximize your time to squeeze in reading. During lunch or break time at work, you can scan a publication and flag longer articles to read later when you have more time or can concentrate better. Perhaps you can schedule a thirty-minute block of time either before or after your shift to catch up on some reading or an online class. You may feel that you work enough hours already, and you probably do, but pursuing continuing education should be considered part of your job. It is just not forced upon you during the hours you are obligated to your employer. Always keep a journal or two on hand, in your satchel or in your car, to read during unexpected waits. Even ten minutes can get you through a good continuing education article while you're waiting in line at the post office or grocery store. When you are visiting a doctor yourself, or taking your kids to the dentist, bring along a few journals. You will undoubtedly have time to read. If you have a long commute back and forth to work in the car or have a road trip planned, purchase conference proceedings or educational materials on CD. This is a great time to do more than gaze through the windshield and hum along with the radio. If you're traveling on a plane, there will be lots of time to read educational material, rather than tabloid magazines. When you look closely at your daily or weekly routine, you probably have more down time than you realize. The trick is to always, always, have at least one or two publications on your person at all times, and get creative about other ways to soak in information.

6

STAFF COMMUNICATION

The veterinary team is only as good as the communication between its members. No one on the team can care for a patient or client all alone, not even the veterinarian, so effort must be made to constantly improve and monitor the communication in your practice. This can be difficult, to say the least. All of us have individual personalities, and we have different communication styles. Some people are abrupt and are not good at sugar-coating their comments; others need to be handled more gently and get offended easily; and some tend to become angry and defensive when confronted with differing opinions It is the mixture of personalities that can make it difficult to communicate, but that mixture is also what makes a great team. What one person lacks, another makes up for, and so there is a balance and compliment of styles. This chapter is a discussion of communication and how it can be improved in your practice.

What is the best way for me to enhance communication between the front office and the medical staff?

Even though many practices are physically separated into front and back working areas, the best practices do not have this separation between the different team members in each area. It's important that communication flow freely and constantly between the front and the back of a practice.

In order to ensure the flow of information, it is important to develop systems and protocols that address how and when communication should occur so everyone knows what to expect. For example, the front office team knows not to check out a client until the technician has either come up with the client or called on the phone to let the front office know that the client is ready to go. When an unusual situation occurs, communicate it immediately by leaving notes for each other or using a dry-erase board that is centrally located near the workstations. Check in with each other often during the day, so everyone has the same information. During staff meetings, ensure that each area has a chance to contribute on issues that affect the entire practice. It can help when each area has a supervisor or lead person who can help to distribute information and express opinions when there are issues.

All of these tactical approaches are good for opening up the lines of communication, but attitude, courtesy, and mutual respect are key ingredients in front-to-back conversation. Each group should appreciate the other's position in the practice. This is often accomplished by cross-training and helping out in the other area when needed. Role playing and role reversal can also be good tools to use during training and team building. The staff should appreciate each other as people outside of their position in the practice, so be sure to involve all team members in outside events. Finally, expressing appreciation for all positive contributions is essential to creating harmony throughout the practice and making communication flow easier.

How can I improve communication between the veterinarians and the technicians?

Our patients depend on good communication between all members of the veterinary team, particularly the veterinarians and technicians. For general issues affecting the medical team, it is helpful to have structured communication events in the practice, such as routine staff meetings or departmental meetings to discuss more specific topics. An internal staff newsletter can be a great source of general information, and each subgroup can have its own space devoted to its members: front office staff, technicians, assistants, veterinarians, etc. This newsletter can be printed, posted, and distributed, or it can be delivered via e-mail. Interoffice e-mail can be another method for communicating when there isn't time for the team to meet physically.

Off-duty staff can get caught up with changes when they come back to work if you designate that e-mail inboxes need to be checked at the beginning of each shift; that time should be part of the paid shift on the clock. Be certain that the e-mail policy is addressed in the employee handbook and that everyone knows the rules. Be careful not to e-mail an important request or vital information, since you cannot count on when the message will be received.

There is no substitute for face-to-face communication when the topic involves patients in our care, or issues that may be sensitive or timely. Patients in the hospital should be discussed each morning. The medical staff should gather to review every patient at the beginning of the day and repeat this process in the afternoon in a twenty-four-hour practice. The patient's treatment can be reviewed, progress discussed, and any upcoming procedures or diagnostics planned.

In order for good communication to occur, about patients and otherwise, there needs to be mutual respect between team members. Training that brings together members of the medical staff can help establish and enhance mutual respect, as each staff member understands what the other people in the group have to learn and contribute.

Veterinarians should participate in the training of technicians, and both should present in-house continuing education events that the other group attends. It also helps to have social activities or more lighthearted events that bring together the veterinarians and technicians. There are times when the medical hierarchy can get in the way, but everyone deserves to be treated with respect regardless of his or her credentials. Stepping away from the practice can help the team see each other as people first and professionals second. This can enhance everyone's willingness to communicate in a respectful way.

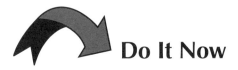 **Do It Now**

Set up interoffice e-mail for all employees on the team, with a detailed policy of use established in the employee handbook and explained to the entire team.

How can I motivate employees to work as a team?

Every team has to work toward a mutually agreed-upon goal. So the first method of motivating your team is to refocus on the mission or goal of the practice. For your subsection of employees, your objective may be to provide excellent patient care and treat every pet as if it were your own. Sometimes employees need to be reminded of how their daily tasks contribute to this bigger objective. A squabble between employees disrupts the flow of information between them, which can result in diminished care for the patient.

When a team member is consistently late, patient treatments are delayed. When one person is having a bad day and not putting his or her effort into work, attention to detail falls to the wayside. Mistakes can be made in calculating medication doses, administering treatments, or performing procedures. The team has to remain focused on the ultimate goal and support each other in that effort. There is a larger team in the practice that includes the entire staff. In order to support the entire team, it is important to understand and appreciate everyone's position. This appreciation can be accomplished with cross-training and job swapping. Since cross-training and job rotation can get pushed to the side when things get busy, it is important to work job swaps into the staff schedule routinely, to strengthen the team.

The team should remain energized and cohesive by attending staff meetings where each area of the practice is represented (front office, assistants, technician staff, veterinarians, etc.) and open discussion is encouraged. There should be no hierarchy when it comes to mutual respect, and everyone should be expected to contribute to and do the dirty work when needed. This helps each team member to feel important and see that his or her contribution is important.

You can plan activities outside of work to bring the team together without the normal stresses of the job, so the team members can form relationships on a different level. When team members know each other better, it is easier for them to communicate openly about good and bad issues as the workday progresses. Lastly, remember that a team is made up of individuals, and each person wants and needs to feel recognized and appreciated. Say thank you to each other often, and expect the same from the owner and leadership team.

RESOURCES
Teams That Work (CD-ROM), by Mary Ann Vande Linde, DVM (Lifelearn 2004)

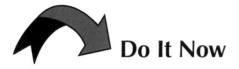

Do It Now

Help your team develop a job-swapping
schedule so that everyone can pitch in
where needed when the work needs
to get done! Determine the slower days
of the week when this swap will be most
appropriate, and write the swaps actually
on to the work schedules of the team
so that staff members are prepared
when the day comes.

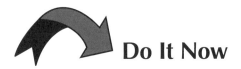 **Do It Now**

Help your team to create a schedule of
events outside of work so they can bring
that positive energy back into work and
be more efficient. These events can
include a picnic, a barbecue, going to
a movie, visiting a local zoo or botanical
garden, playing a team sport, taking
a bike ride or hike, or having a theme party.
Gather ideas from the entire team
so everyone's wishes are considered.
Make the schedule out for the year
so everyone has these events
to look forward to.

What is the best way for us to alert the rest of the staff that an emergency patient is in transit to the practice?

When a client or referring practice calls ahead, everyone on the team needs to know that a critical patient is in transit. Even in a smaller practice, there are staff members who may not be within hearing distance if this patient's expected arrival is only announced verbally. There are many things that can happen between hanging up the phone with the caller and the arrival of the patient, such as shift changes, lunch breaks, or rotation of employees. A consistent communication system should be used in these circumstances.

The front office staff will be the first to see the patient arrive, so they need a system of communication for their team. A small white board at the main greeting station (the one centrally located, closest to the door, that receives the most client traffic) can be filled out. This white board should not be in the view of clients. It should contain the name of the client and patient on the way, species/breed, and type of crisis. Then everyone up front knows to expect a bulldog named Lucky Jones who is having trouble breathing, and they will see that he receives immediate attention upon arrival.

There should be a standard protocol for the client's arrival depending on the type of crisis. For this emergency involving breathing difficulty, the front office staff should know that they need to take the pet immediately to the back treatment area for respiratory support. Perhaps in another situation, the front office staff will escort the client and patient to an exam room, or call for a triage in the lobby first.

The medical staff will be ready for Lucky as well. Create a more detailed triage board in the back treatment area, in a location that is visible to the majority of the medical staff. The information on the board will include the client and patient name, species, breed, age, sex, type of crisis, and estimated time of arrival. The technicians on duty in this main treatment area should remain vigilant of this board and keep the attending veterinarians informed as well. They should have supplies and equipment waiting to assist the patient in trouble. For Lucky's arrival, the "crash cart" and oxygen supply are ready to go!

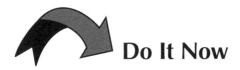 **Do It Now**

Buy two wet- or dry-erase boards,
one smaller and one relatively large.
Buy some black or colored striping tape.
Create an emergency board in front,
and a triage board in back, so everyone
can move quickly when a patient
in crisis arrives. Include the appropriate
columns for necessary information:
client name, patient name, signalment
(breed/species/gender/age), presenting
problem, estimated time of arrival,
and assigned doctor for the case.

How can we react efficiently when a patient is experiencing an emergency?

A "crash" event is one of those occasions that should be part of routine and repeated team training. All persons or positions have jobs to do, and they need to know their tasks and feel comfortable whether they perform them once a day, once a week, or just every once in a while. In fact, the less often your practice sees emergency patients, the more often you should conduct routine team training and mock drills. To develop this training plan, determine all the necessary functions that need to occur during a crash, and assign each duty to a particular position (not necessarily to a specific person, because the staff changes depending on the shift, time of day, day of the week, etc.). Everyone should know their part so that nothing is left out and people are not falling over each other trying to do the same tasks.

There should be a sporadic, scheduled, but unexpected calendar of mock crash drills. At varying times and days of the week, someone can initiate the crash drill by using a stuffed animal dummy. A front office person can call back a fake triage for the board, then come running back to the treatment area at the estimated time of arrival with the stuffed patient. There are times when patients in crisis arrive without forewarning, so there should be times when the stuffed patient in crisis is just rushed to the back without advanced notice. There needs to be an assigned technician and/or veterinarian on board with the drill to yell out the patient's status and problem as if it were really happening.

This scenario should be altered at each drill to represent different types of emergencies. To represent an in-hospital patient emergency, a technician or veterinarian can be assigned to initiate the drill with the stuffed patient that has been sneaked into a cage or run, and then "discovered" by the assigned person. Once the event begins, everyone should go through all the appropriate motions. One team member, perhaps a member of management, should stand back and observe, recording the strengths and weaknesses of the drill and of individual performances. When the crisis has passed, the team should immediately discuss any issues that were experienced and decide how to improve their teamwork. It is much better to learn during these exercises than to make mistakes during a real crisis when moments count and a patient is counting on you!

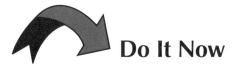 **Do It Now**

Together with the team, designate crash assignments so that everyone knows their part during a crisis. With the management team, develop a schedule of unexpected mock crash training drills, and determine who will initiate the drill and who will observe to assess the success of the participants.

How can I communicate ongoing patient needs to all the staff?

E very patient in the hospital has specific needs, whether the animal is staying for an hour, an afternoon, or an extended period of time. The only way each patient will receive the necessary care is through good team communication. There are multiple ways to communicate patient instructions. Often, the method depends on the size of the practice, the layout of the facility, and the number of staff available at any given time. Depending on these factors, there will be necessary repetition of information as well.

Alerts regarding medical conditions or cautions should be easily visible with bright stickers or colored markers near the patient on a cage card. These should also be placed on treatment sheets or boards. A treatment sheet can be hung directly on the cage for each patient, but in smaller cages this can interfere with visibility of the patient. Therefore, a central location for treatment sheets can be used. Dry-erase boards can be helpful in tracking the overall needs of patients in a certain area. These boards can be sectioned off with black tape, with individual patient names along the top and hour segments along the side. In the box with the appropriate time, you can note when to feed, walk, or medicate a patient. The instructions, however, will not be followed just because the note is posted. There should be staff assigned to a group of patients or an area of the hospital, and it is this person's responsibility to perform the patient care tasks. This staff person will ensure that the treatment sheet or board is updated regularly, and she will inform additional staff of the patient needs at shift change or before time away from the floor. The assigned person is also the go-to person for the veterinarian to obtain information about the patient's progress.

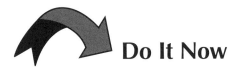 **Do It Now**

Buy a large wet- or dry-erase board,
markers, erasers, and black or colored
striping tape. Create a white board for the
patient care area that will guide patient
treatments. Create a column for each
cage represented in the area and
a row for each of twelve hours
(a.m. and p.m. will be designated
on the specific order).

What is the best way for us to keep track of patients' belongings during their stay?

It is difficult to refuse all pet possessions, because the family is looking for ways to comfort their beloved pet. However, it is fine to limit the number of items that you are talked into keeping. Assure the client that his pet will be given soft bedding and kept warm and comfortable. Let him know that toys are not generally appropriate for a hospitalized patient. The easiest way to prevent keeping leashes and collars is to have a supply of hospital leashes on hand at all times to switch with the clients' leashes and collars.

If items are stored at the hospital, they need to be clearly marked in a non-permanent manner. White bandage tape or masking tape and a Sharpie black felt-tip pen works fine for toys and other items. Pet carriers can also be marked in this way, but you might consider something more appealing, such as nice tags or labels, since clients often keep a carrier marked. If the items are to be used by the pet, and subsequently laundered, then you'll need to find a more robust method of marking, such as plastic "price tags" that are hooked onto the item, or safety-pinned bits of marked cloth. Even if the item is marked, a description of the item should appear on the patient's treatment sheet or medical record. The item needs to be stored in a location that is known by the entire team, is consistent for patients in that area or section, and can easily accommodate the size or type of items left.

For smaller items, an organizer bag with multiple pockets can be clipped onto or near the cage that can hold possessions and additional medications or supplies. You can even make your own low-cost pouches by cutting the tops off used fluid bags and hanging those on the cage. Another method is to place the smaller items in a plastic, sealable bag with their name marked clearly, and store the bags in a cabinet, storage drawers, or shelving system that is specified for that purpose. The drawers can be marked alphabetically to help the search. You may have space available for separate baskets that can be assigned to a patient. If it comforts the family to leave an item, try to accommodate them, with the appropriate disclaimer that the practice cannot be held liable for return or condition of the items.

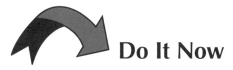 **Do It Now**

Create a task force with a representative
from each area: front office, technician
team, assistant or kennel staff,
and a member of management.
Have a team meeting to discuss the best
method of organizing patient belongings,
and assign action steps and a deadline to
see the project to completion.
Train the entire team on the use of the
system, and reevaluate the success of the
system at one-month, three-month,
and six-month intervals.
Make adjustments as necessary.

How can we be sure to remember to return outside radiograph films to the client or original practice?

It is important to realize that original radiographs are part of a patient's permanent medical record, and these films belong to the practice that performed the radiography. Therefore, the films need to be tracked within your practice so they can be returned promptly. Radiographs should be logged into a manual or computerized system. The information should include the client and patient name, original practice and veterinarian, number of films received, and the date and staff member who received them. When they are mailed back or returned to the client, this return date and method, and the staff member involved, will be added to this log. If a practice management software system is used, it is often possible to create a flag, block, or notice that will pop up to remind the staff that radiographs arrived with this patient. Otherwise, the hard copy of the patient's chart should be flagged. The radiograph sleeve or envelope should be tagged as well, preferably with a removable note or card so it can be taken off upon release back to the client.

While the radiographs remain in the practice, there should be central locations for these films. This can be in the doctors' area so they have access to the films during the patient's stay, or somewhere near the patient areas. When the patient is ready for discharge, a flag on the medical record will prompt the team to locate the radiographs and return them to the client. If needed, the films can be mailed back to the original veterinarian in a timely fashion. There should be a protocol that assigns a team member and follows a consistent mailing schedule. If your practice is releasing original films to clients, this transfer needs to be documented so you can follow up with the client and/or referral practice for return of the films. As mentioned, they are part of your patient's medical record, and you need to retain these records for the amount of time prescribed by your state for retention of patient records.

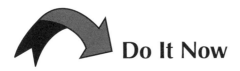 ## Do It Now

Create a task force with a representative from each area: front office, technician team, assistant or kennel staff, and a member of management. Have a team meeting to discuss the best method of organizing outside radiographs, and assign action steps and a deadline to see the project to completion. Train the entire team on the use of the system, and reevaluate the success of the system at one-month, three-month, and six-month intervals. Make adjustments as necessary.

7

WORK FLOW

The purpose of establishing good work flow protocols is to keep the work flowing! There is usually no shortage of work, even when the patient load is light. There are always things that need to be done, such as stocking, cleaning, organizing, and other assorted projects. When the practice is busy with incoming clients and patients, it is important to prioritize tasks and be able to juggle multiple things at the same time. There are times when you must also juggle multiple doctors, anticipating what each one needs as you move through the day. There are even times when you need to be able to get the doctors moving forward from one examination room to the next. Patient appointments need to be scheduled efficiently, as well as team members, to get the work done within the scheduled hours. There are no shortages of challenges when it comes to work flow in the veterinary practice.

How do I manage my time when everyone wants everything from me yesterday? How can I make people understand that I can't do everything for everyone all the time?

First you need to know what the main responsibilities are for your position, so you can prioritize effectively. If you have a job description, use this as your starting point. As requests come up that are not spelled out clearly in your job description, go to your supervisor or manager. Lay out your current duties and projects, and ask for their help in prioritizing the list. It is important to find out what your management team views as your top priorities.

If it seems that everyone wants something from you "yesterday," then an anticipated deadline is not being communicated. Get in the habit of asking the person how soon they expect the task to be performed. If they need it done now, and you cannot give their task first priority, then explain the reason for the delay and see if someone else needs to be delegated the task. Then realize that no, you can't do everything for everyone, all of the time. This is when respectful, effective communication is needed. Acknowledge the request and the importance of the expectation. Clearly state what you can and cannot do for that person, and the time period in which you can deliver on his or her request. Give a brief explanation of what you are actually doing and why you can't change the priority of your tasks at the very moment. Typically, the reason would involve patient needs, or the top spot on your list has already been spoken for.

Try to have an alternative solution to offer, such as giving him or her a time line when you can get the task performed, or offering to ask someone else on the team who may be available at the time. It's all about communication, and how to avoid feeling squeezed from all sides.

How can I stay cool and calm when frustrations come up during a busy day? Even when I feel I am doing my best, situations pop up that are not under my control.

Although this is typical for our profession, it can also be frustrating and overwhelming at times. Realize that while situations are often beyond your control, the way you react to them is totally in your control, and you're not alone. Good communication helps the team get through a rough patch together. Keep everyone informed about what is going on, especially between the front office and the back treatment area. Often these two areas are experiencing completely different levels of work and chaos at any given time. So it's important to communicate and be able to step in to another area to help when needed, or expect their help in return. Members of the management team can also pitch in where needed, as long as they are informed of the need. Many managers or supervisors start out as front office team members or technicians, so they have not lost those skills when they gained a desk.

It is also helpful for the management team members to observe the staff handling chaos and crisis, to help them assess performance and future practice needs. Communicate with clients as well, or else you will have to add dealing with client confrontations to your list of duties. Let them know of any expected wait times, and the reasons for the wait if the length of time is extensive (typically over fifteen minutes). You may need the front office staff to communicate the wait time to the clients out in the lobby. This is when cross-training is most valuable, and the front office can learn how to discharge patients, provide routine restraint, or fill medications depending on your practice's policies.

When the front office is crazy, be willing to come up and help address some of the client needs or answer the phone. Do not always wait to be asked; if you are keeping your eyes open to the flow of the work, you will notice when your help might be needed.

Most important, do not panic, and try to help others to avoid the same. Take a deep breath, divert the crisis-mentality of the team by providing encouragement and humor, and all of you will reach the end of the shift, eventually.

How do I learn to better anticipate the doctors' needs?

Start by asking the doctor you work with most often, and explain to her that you want to better anticipate her needs. Ask her to explain her thought process as she works through an appointment, procedure, or surgery. If she just verbalizes her thoughts, it will help you learn what she wants next and needs from you in particular. Start the appointment, procedure, or surgery by asking her what supplies she will need so you can gather them together and have them readily available. In addition, during the event, be observant and watch what the doctor asks for next. Keep a small notebook and pen in your pocket, and take notes during this observation if you are able. If it is not appropriate to stop and write at that time, try to take a minute after the event to jot down a few notes that you recall. If you simply outline the flow of events, it will give you something to review later.

Go over your notes with the doctor at a later time, if possible. This will demonstrate to the doctor that you are committed to being an asset to her, and she will be more willing to help with the process. Next time you perform the same procedure with the same doctor, follow your notes to see if you need to change or add any details. You may want to keep a separate small notebook for each doctor, or each type of procedure, depending on your preference.

In the hectic reality that is daily life in the veterinary practice, it may be unlikely that you can stop and take notes. In this case, consider asking your manager or owner if you can come in on your day off to shadow a doctor and technician as they perform their daily tasks. Choose the doctor you work with most often, when she is paired with a technician you know to be a star performer. Ask your manager or owner if you need help choosing the best mentor technician and the best day to shadow. Take notes as the doctor and the technician move along, and use these outlines as a starting point later when you're on the clock.

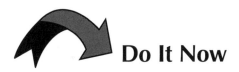 **Do It Now**

Keep a small notepad and mini or
telescopic pen in your pocket at all times to
take notes and stay organized.
Use it regularly!

What is the most efficient way of scheduling appointments?

You may be able to prioritize according to patient need to make your schedule more efficient, such as giving time slots first thing in the morning and following the lunch period with animals that are ill or injured so that you have time for diagnostics and lab work by the end of the day. Alternatively, you can schedule all of your compromised patients in the morning, so procedures or surgeries can take place midday to allow for patient recovery in the afternoon. Routine wellness visits may be scheduled during these afternoons.

In practices that perform multiple routine surgeries such as spays and neuters, there can either be blocks of time each day, or multiple entire days, set aside for these surgeries. The appointment schedule should also include blocks of unscheduled time that are used as a buffer when things run late or unexpected emergencies have to be worked in. Typically, a buffer will be scheduled midmorning, midday, and midafternoon. Although the appointment schedule should be pre-set so that clients can anticipate your hours, there still needs to be some flexibility within those operating hours. Specific clients who routinely require more time can be scheduled longer, or you can schedule multiple appointment slots. It is important to communicate to all the staff members who schedule appointments which clients need extra time. There are specific patients who may require a longer appointment, particularly if you can anticipate what treatment or procedure they will need during the visit. Develop a list of these red-flagged appointment types for the front office staff training, such as requested clip-nails-express-anal-glands-annual-vaccinations combos, skin problems, behavior issues, or sick visits. The most efficient schedule is one where clients do not wait long on average, and no patient is ever turned away.

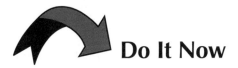 **Do It Now**

Schedule a buffer time slot in your
appointment schedule to allow for
catch-up time. There may be a need
for a buffer slot in the morning,
and one in the afternoon. Evaluate the
success of this system at regular intervals,
and adjust as necessary.

How can we schedule employees
more effectively?

Once you are operating on a set appointment schedule, you can compare the revenue generated each day with the amount of money spent on staffing. Knowing the overall budget for payroll, you will gain an idea of how much staff you can afford to have on any given day based on seasonal and weekly trends. Beyond the financial considerations, there are many options for scheduling staff. You may only be responsible for scheduling the technician team, based on the overall needs of the practice. It's important to involve the staff members as much as possible. Explain that you will not be able to accommodate everyone's desires, but you want collective input on how they think the schedule can be more efficient. Typically, the team working that schedule knows a great deal about positive changes that can be implemented; they just need to be asked. Instead of asking, "When do you want to work?" ask questions that guide the larger discussion. Depending on the operating hours of your practice, you may have the team consider eight-, ten-, or twelve-hour shifts. Guide the team in a discussion of how to block the schedule; for example, days working in a row and days off in a row. Weekends are usually another topic of discussion, and a fair solution needs to have everyone rotating in on the weekends. Remember to discuss holiday schedules as well. There needs to be a fair way to rotate holidays so that everyone has a chance to spend a holiday with his or her family. It may not be the same holiday every year, but people in veterinary medicine typically understand that pets do not simply stay well on holidays for our convenience.

Aside from these big questions, there are smaller ones that need to be addressed. When there are shift changes, plan for an overlap to allow for rounding on patients. With longer shifts especially, be sure that there are scheduled lunch and break times to help the employees maintain their stamina.

When discussing efficiency, there are two ways to look at the employee schedule. First, the end result should be an employee schedule that achieves excellent patient and client care with the minimum number of staff. Second, all team members should perform their duties in an organized and capable manner. If the employee schedule does not seem to be efficient, analyze the number of people required to get the job done, but do not neglect to consider the work result of each individual on the team.

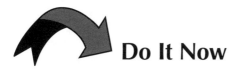 **Do It Now**

Hold a team meeting to discuss the
current employee schedule, and welcome
discussion on any suggested changes based
on client needs and employee preferences.
Be sure that management is represented
at this meeting; any changes need to be
agreed upon by the majority of the team.
Reevaluate success of the
new schedule at regular intervals.

How do I teach doctors and staff to better budget their time, so they aren't always running late and working overtime?

For the most part, no one wants overtime. You and your team members put in long days already, and the last thing you want to see at the end of a grueling shift is another hour of work ahead of you. But if you don't know why you're running into overtime, it will never go away. One way to examine this issue is through time management analysis. When you look back at a busy day, it's all a blur and you're not sure why you find yourself running into overtime at the end of it. There are two ways to dissect your day and find some answers. First, you can create a time log of events and track what you do during the day. This requires time itself, however, and complete honesty. Because each day is different, this exercise should be done for a week straight.

If you have management's support, they could allow you the option of confidential analysis. This means that you collect the data, you analyze where you are spending your time, and you commit to making some changes. You don't have to share every moment of your day with your manager, so you can't be chastised for a personal phone call or occasional chitchats. The other option is to have someone else track you, but this has disadvantages. For one, if someone is watching over your shoulder, you are likely to perform your duties differently and be more effective during the day for the simple reason that someone is watching you. You won't sneak off for that personal call, or stop and chat so often. Therefore, this does not necessarily result in an accurate reflection of your day.

If you find yourself overwhelmed with your duties and working overtime on a routine basis, you may want your manager to shadow you so that he or she can help you organize and prioritize your duties. In other words, you are legitimately working as efficiently as possible, and still cannot avoid overtime. You want to prove this to your manager or supervisor, and get his or her advice on how to better prioritize, delegate duties, or distribute the workload. The only way you can learn how to avoid overtime, or be taught by others to work more efficiently, is by knowing where the day is slipping away from you.

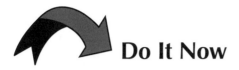 **Do It Now**

Complete a time management analysis,
either performed by a manager or
an employee, to analyze the use of time
each day during a routine week
in practice. Determine where time can
be managed better, and make
changes as needed. Repeat the time management analysis at regular intervals
(every six months) to stay on track
with efficient use of time.

How do I tactfully speed up a veterinarian in the exam room?

If you are fighting the clock despite a good appointment protocol that utilizes the technicians as much as possible, your team may need to develop some scripts, codes, and methods to move things along. When a technician and doctor work together often, the technician develops a sense of how long it should take that doctor to complete that type of appointment, or that phase of the appointment. When that amount of time is up, or the next appointment is ready to be seen, you can use a silent signal such as tapping your wrist watch outside of the client's field of vision if you are in the exam room. If you have previously left the room, you can slip back in to ask if there is anything you can do to help with the client's visit. If there are supplies, educational materials, or products to gather up, these can be delivered to the client at that time and provide the doctor the necessary break in conversation to move toward saying goodbye. If there are still tasks that you need to perform, such as administering medications and performing treatments, enter the room with your supplies and the discussion will be redirected to the next steps of the appointment. If the doctors wear pagers or there is a speaker phone system in each room, a numerical paging code or ring signal can be transmitted that informs them that time is growing short. Or the gold standard is simply peeking in the room to interrupt politely.

Many teams will tell the "white lie" that the doctor is needed in an emergency situation in the back. Be careful about this mistruth, however. Clients become sympathetic or concerned, even if they know it is not their pet experiencing the emergency. They may ask questions of the front desk on their way out, to see how the poor pet is doing. The front office may be put into a sensitive position. At the very least, lying about an emergency is just not necessary. Instead you can say, "Doctor, you are needed in the treatment area" without indicating an emergency situation.

The team should discuss the code phrases you will use, so everyone knows what the hidden meaning is behind the words. Plus, you should discuss together how to help move things along when appointments are getting backed up. Often the veterinarian wants to be "rescued" from the exam room as well, so she will welcome your polite interruption. Even if the veterinarian chooses to stay an extra moment to finish up and say goodbye, you have at least made her aware of the time.

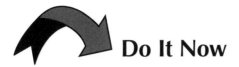 **Do It Now**

Develop a private code for your team to move doctors along in the exam room. This should be a simple phrase that is nonchalant and not obvious to the client, so that it seems to be part of the routine: "Doctor, would you like for me to 1) take Fido out for a walk now? 2) put Fluffy back in her carrier?" as if the appointment is wrapping up, for example.

How do I handle a doctor
who is always running late?

This can be a difficult scenario, and there are many factors that could be contributing. If the doctor is consistently getting stuck longer in exam rooms than your appointment schedule allows, then it might be time to re-think the appointment schedule. First you need to answer the question: Is the doctor too chatty, or just moving slowly? Is the conversation focused entirely on the client and his pet's needs, so that the time is invested in great client service, or does the doctor allow herself to be drawn off topic, into other areas that may not enhance the mission of the practice?

When adjusting the appointment schedule to fit in more time per client, the practice sees fewer appointments. However, if the clients that are spending longer with that doctor tend to spend more money and take better care of their pets, then it may be well worth that additional appointment time. Perhaps your doctor is consistently behind with procedures or in-hospital patients that are left waiting. This will require better communication about when patients should be anesthetized or prepared for a pending procedure or adding a buffer time in a crammed surgery schedule.

Rather than focusing on the doctor as the problem, it may be necessary to step back and analyze the flow of work in the practice to identify where improvements can be made for the benefit of the clients with appointments, the patients needing attention, and the staff members who are waiting in the wings.

How can I bounce between multiple veterinarians and efficiently assist them during daily activities?

When first learning how to juggle multiple doctors, or when a new doctor joins the mix, rely heavily on taking notes. Keep a notepad and pen in your pocket at all times, and do not hesitate to write down tips and tasks along the way. Note preferences of each individual doctor. Keep a running to-do list as you move through the day. Constantly reprioritize the items on your list. Learn to triage your doctors' requests just as they learn to triage their patients. Time-sensitive, critical issues come first. Then move on to those issues that will become bigger issues if not handled soon, and finally those issues that should be addressed but are not time sensitive.

You also need to learn how to delegate to assistants and other technicians. The most important tip in delegation is this: Always *ask* your team members to help, never *tell* them. On the flip side, when you're asked for help by a veterinarian or coworker, you need to be honest about your current workload. If at all possible, jump in and help. But if you're already working on your own to-do list and are involved in a high-priority item, be honest about what you can do for others. If you've agreed to help or complete a request, then stay in touch with the person who requested it of you. Update this person on your availability status, and remind her that you haven't forgotten the request.

If at all possible in your practice, it is helpful to assign a technician to each doctor on duty. This gives the doctor a go-to person, and each technician has to work mainly with one doctor consistently, at least during that shift. It can provide for much smoother client and patient care as well. The family comes to know that doctor-technician team, and the patient is being cared for consistently by the same few people all day long. You will need to account for overlap, however. What happens when a patient needs to be anesthetized while the doctor is finishing up an appointment? Perhaps you have a surgery or pre-op technician who handles those functions for all the doctors on duty. This also works in other areas of the practice such as the in-house laboratory. It's the equivalent of having a combination of one-to-one and zone coverage.

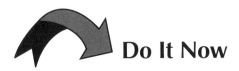 **Do It Now**

Purchase a small notebook and mini-pen or lanyard pen for every staff member to keep handy. When starting this notebook system, the person who fills up her notebook first could get a fun reward to keep the positive momentum.

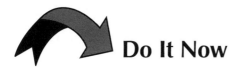 **Do It Now**

Assign a technician to a specific doctor,
and assign a technician to a hospital
zone or area. Be certain to involve
management and the doctors in the
decision of who to pair together
and where to assign different technicians,
based on their personality mix
and skill sets.

How am I able to get small projects done that my boss wants me to do, and still do my job full time in a busy clinic?

The short answer is this: If your boss wants it done, he or she needs to give you time to do it. The long answer, however, is more complicated. There are probably a handful of projects and assignments that you are trying to juggle, along with patient and client care. Are there too many for you to handle, and can you accept more assignments? You will only know if you track what you've already committed to doing. Keep a running list of all your projects, and update it when necessary. For each project, summarize the goal, outline the tasks involved, and estimate the amount of time it will take to complete. This will result in an estimated completion date. The management team may have assigned a deadline when you accepted the project. If not, be sure you ask when they expect it to be completed, and discuss a realistic time frame, taking into consideration your other projects and main position duties. If you have multiple projects, then you may need their help in assigning or rearranging priorities.

Each time you're able to work on this project, update your project log with the date and length of time you spent. If you see that your deadline or estimated completion date needs to be revised, talk with the owner, manager, or supervisor who assigned the task. It's important to have this project log to review with your management team. Then, if they need the assignment completed, you can demonstrate how much time your current job duties have allowed you to work on it.

If needed, you can justify a request for administrative time off the floor to dedicate to the project. It is unrealistic in most cases to expect technicians to be able to work on a project of any proportion during the down times or slow periods of their regularly scheduled workload, yet this is often what the management team expects. In order to request administrative time, you may have to prove that you cannot possibly accomplish the task during these random slow moments. When it is a project that takes concentration and mental effort, it will be difficult to make progress in between patient and client interruptions. Technicians will always make main duties their top priority, unless they are given specific times and deadlines for getting projects done. Be sure to keep this project log handy for evaluation time too!

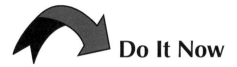

Do It Now

Create a project log to keep your work flowing on these extra assignments. Buy a notebook from an office or school supply store, and document the project name, the date it was assigned, who assigned the project, and the expected due date. Leave enough room between project entries to note each date you work on the project and for how long, and any check-in dates before the due date.

8

SAFETY AND REGULATION

There are laws and regulations that affect what we do every day. Most of these regulations dictate safety rules, such as Occupational Health and Safety Administration (OSHA) guidelines. It's easy to believe that OSHA rules should be followed to keep the practice out of trouble, but the truth is that they are followed to keep you and your colleagues safe each day on the job. The management team can and should enforce these safety rules, and adherence to these policies is part of your job performance. We should all be smart while doing the physical work our jobs require, so that none of us suffers adverse effects from our years in this career. A clean environment is also a safe environment, and every one must do their part to keep the facility well maintained. Our practices often contain controlled substances as well, and there are regulations that need to be followed to avoid dangerous misuse of these drugs. Staying up-to-date on all of these regulations can be challenging, and it takes a team effort.

How can we keep the facility clean and well maintained?

A portion of every technician's job involves keeping the facility clean. Cleanliness is an important aspect of client perception. Clients' initial reaction to your practice will be affected by their experience when they enter the practice and spend time waiting in different locations. To gain the client's perspective, enter your building several times a week from the client entrance. Look around as you enter, and see what your clients see, smell, and hear.

Cleanliness also helps to maintain a safe environment for employees. Keeping the practice clean must be a team effort, and everyone has to do their share no matter what their credentials, job title, or seniority.

It is easy to become immune to the clutter that can occur in a veterinary practice, but this clutter can be dangerous when people need to move fast for a critical patient or sudden evacuation. It is important that everything have an assigned place, and this location should be properly labeled for quick reference. Cabinet doors and drawers can be labeled with a list of everything inside. It is much easier to keep the facility clean as you are working. After procedures or treatments, the area and equipment should be cleaned immediately. Cleaning checklists are essential, including various tasks that need to be done in every area of the practice. These checklists should outline daily, weekly, and monthly tasks for each area.

Equipment must be kept safe and working properly as well. To ensure that equipment is routinely serviced, create a system in the computer to generate automatic reminders, or make a chart for each area outlining the service needed. The task can be checked off when completed.

There are always larger cleaning projects that can be tackled during slow periods in the practice. Each area should have a downtime or project list. If these are tasks that need to be done on a routine basis, whether or not there is a long enough slow period, then the projects should be assigned rather than ignored until the next slow period. The entire team should take pride in their environment and keep it safe for each other.

How can we reduce the noise level in the patient boarding areas?

Noise is a hazard that all veterinary professionals face. In a patient boarding or hospitalization area, noise also adversely affects the patients under our care. Every effort should be made to engineer patient areas with materials that reduce echo or amplification. These measures should be considered when building a new facility or addition to the building, but some materials can be added to an existing area to help reduce or absorb environmental noise.

The best relief from noise is to eliminate the noise itself. Typically the worst offenders are our canine patients. When one of them starts barking the chorus begins! There are a few tricks that can quiet down the gang. Music is a good way to soothe man and beast alike, and classical music in particular can keep the dogs' attention quite well. To reduce stress in your patients you can also use systems that release synthetic pheromones into the air continually.

Realize that your patients may be trying to tell you something, and their barks may be more than mere background noise. Increasing the frequency of walks—for example, to four times daily—can help keep the pets more comfortable and quiet. Noise is not only produced from stress, but can cause stress as well. This is true for you and your patients.

Keep in mind that species that are more sensitive to noise and fragile by nature should be located in isolated, quiet areas of the hospital. If at all possible, cats should not be kept near dogs, and exotics need to be kept in their own areas as well. Everyone deserves downtime, even your patients, so plan to turn off the lights and give them quiet time when possible. In a twenty-four-hour practice, we often forget that as fresh employees come on shift, our patients have been exposed to noise and light throughout all those shifts. Give them the "nighttime" that they are used to from their home life. When scheduling treatments or work to be performed in the patient areas, try to bundle the tasks so that you are not constantly disturbing the group and causing chaos. Constant movement in and out of the area will stimulate more of a ruckus and produce more noise.

What is the best way for me to help maintain OSHA compliance in our practice?

Safety should be incorporated into every phase of training. When it's your turn to train new employees, be sure you know the safety rules you are supposed to teach. Also be sure you are setting a good example by following them yourself, both for new hires and in front of the entire team.

If you notice someone violating the safety rules of your practice, try the direct approach first. For example, if you notice someone is not wearing personal protective equipment such as lead aprons in radiology, gently point out that the aprons are provided for his or her safety. Repeat violations should be reported to a member of management. This may be the only way to protect your fellow workers, even from themselves.

The entire team should receive training sessions or a refresher course on an OSHA topic at each staff meeting. If you've noticed that there is a specific problem with safety lately—for example, clutter keeps accumulating in the hallways—mention that topic to your manager prior to the meeting so that it may be considered for the topic of the month. On a daily basis, safety hazards should be reported to management immediately to be corrected.

If you take an interest in safety, offer to become the safety officer or assist the current officer in his or her duties. The safety officer position needs to be recognized by the management team with a separate job description and compensation consideration. This person needs to be given the authority to correct unsafe conditions and employee actions. On a monthly basis, mock inspections should be performed by the safety officer to note any dangerous conditions or things that need to be repaired or replaced. The officer can also be the person to address the team at staff meetings, take charge of initial training of new employees, maintain documentation of employee training, and deliver continuing education on safety topics. Even if you are not interested in going quite this far with your involvement, you can help by keeping your eyes open, knowing your practice's safety rules and protocols, and reporting unsafe conditions so that you and your coworkers will remain safe.

Keep in mind that OSHA maintains safety in occupations beyond veterinary medicine, so information gained directly from OSHA may need some extrapolating for its application in veterinary medicine. Fortunately, there are several veterinary OSHA consultants who provide information for our profession.

RESOURCES

Be Safe! Veterinary Safety Training for the Medical and Technical Staff, by Phillip J. Seibert, Jr., CVT (AAHA Press 2007)

Be Safe! Veterinary Safety Training for the Whole Practice Team, by Philip J. Seibert, Jr., CVT (AAHA Press 2007)

The Complete Veterinary Practice Regulatory Compliance Manual, Fifth Edition, by Philip J. Seibert, Jr., CVT (Veterinary Practice Consultants 2003)

Safety Handbook for Veterinary Hospital Staff, by Diane McKelvey, DVM (AAHA Press 1999)

Safety in the Veterinary Practice (CD-ROM), by Brian Hayden and George Miller (Lifelearn 2000)

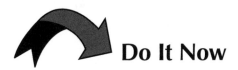 **Do It Now**

Subscribe to the OSHA newsletter
available at www.osha.gov, or find
links to state-specific OSHA news.
Also subscribe to veterinary-specific
OSHA newsletters at www.safetyvet.com
or www.kendricktechservices.com.
This saves time trying
to research compliance.

How can we avoid on-the-job injuries,
especially as we age? For example,
how can we avoid injuring our hands
and backs? How can we avoid foot
and knee problems from standing and
squatting so much?

It begins with realizing our physical limitations, and not pushing ourselves beyond those limits. Even tasks that do not seem physically taxing can become strenuous, such as prolonged patient restraint. Rotate technicians that are assigned to exam room restraint duty. If you are stuck in a restraint hold for a prolonged period, and you're beginning to feel the physical strain, speak up. Let your doctor know that you need to reposition or switch with another assistant or technician. Always follow safety guidelines for picking up heavy items. Large animals can seem to weigh twice as much as the same weight box with their limbs flailing and bodies folding. Ask for help! Many of you stand on your feet nearly all day long, so invest in supportive footwear that will comfort your feet and protect your back. Your hands are your living, so treat them well also. Wear gloves as needed to prevent the spread of infection, but also to protect your hands from harsh cleaning chemicals and medical solutions. You probably wash your hands dozens of times a day, so use hand cleansers that sanitize but also moisturize, and have a bottle of hand lotion near every sink. Use protective equipment for repetitive duties, such as back braces for heavy lifting. Use equipment that does your work for you such as lift tables. If your duties include activities that you can predict will be strenuous, prepare ahead of time with stretching exercises to stay flexible.

Ergonomic engineering is extremely important in every aspect of your job. Chairs need to be ergonomically designed and raised to the correct height, and counter equipment such as computers and monitors should be positioned correctly. The most important thing is to know your body and to be aware of the warning signs. If you feel fatigue setting in while performing a duty, try to switch out with another team member.

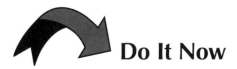 **Do It Now**

Purchase bulk hand lotion at a discount
store and place a dispenser at each sink for
employee use. Refill as needed.
This reduces time spent going to a locker
or purse after every hand washing,
and it protects the employees' hands.

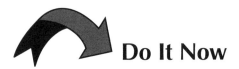

Do It Now

Contact your practice's health insurance provider and inquire about ergonomics training for your staff. Set up this training during a staff meeting or as a mandatory additional meeting for the team.

How do we keep the controlled drug logs accurate and up-to-date with the latest laws and regulations?

You can develop a day log where any surgeries or patients requiring anesthesia are recorded before being logged into the controlled drug book at the end of the day. The day log contains minimal but important information, including the type of controlled drug, the patient/client name and ID number, and the date. It should not take a lot of extra time, but it provides a backup log in case there is a discrepancy discovered in the actual controlled drug logs. It is difficult to trace back on the cases to try to find a missing quantity of controlled drugs by searching the appointment book, or thumbing through medical charts.

At frequent intervals, cross-match the controlled drug logs. Even though the Drug Enforcement Administration (DEA) only requires a physical inventory of controlled substances every two years, most practices inventory these drugs every month. It is even better to perform a quick cross-match on a weekly basis. The sooner a discrepancy is located, the easier it is to rectify. In order to maintain accountability of the system, someone needs to be in charge (or it can be a tag team of several employees or a member of management).

The rules surrounding controlled drugs can also change, and the practice needs to remain aware of current regulations. The most common change occurs with drug classification. Suddenly, a drug that did not need to be recorded requires documentation, so the DEA Web site should be checked frequently.

RESOURCES
Controlled Substance Log, by the American Animal Hospital Association (AAHA Press 2003)
Drug Enforcement Administration (for federal DEA information), www.deadiversion.usdoj. gov

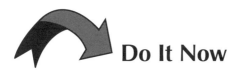 **Do It Now**

Assign the closing or evening technician
to a cross-matching routine for your controlled drugs so that when counts
do not match up, it takes less time
to investigate the error.

How can I stay informed of federal and state regulation changes?

In addition to the OSHA guidelines for general workplace safety and the DEA regulations for controlled drug monitoring, there are federal and state laws, rules, and regulations that can change. These can affect your profession when they describe the duties that you are allowed to do as a credentialed technician in your state. Typically, the attending veterinarian is responsible for facing legal charges brought about by a pet owner, and the technicians and support staff are covered under the doctor's professional liability insurance. However, technicians can be sued for malpractice in some situations and some states, so it is important to stay current on the inherent risks in your job. There are many ways to stay updated, but they do require constant vigilance and effort on your part. To assist with this effort, it is helpful if the practice has a space, such as a bulletin board in an employee area that is dedicated to this type of information. When the management team or employees find updates to post, they can make them available to the entire staff. These topics can also be material for staff or section meetings, or employee newsletters.

Where can you find these updates? By tuning in to the many resources available to technicians and the veterinary profession. The National Association of Veterinary Technicians in America (NAVTA) produces a quarterly magazine that is focused on the veterinary technician profession. The national veterinary association, American Veterinary Medical Association (AVMA), provides information on its Web site regarding animal and public health, as well as updates affecting the profession. Your state's veterinary medical association will keep abreast of federal and state regulation changes that affect the veterinary medicine industry.

RESOURCES
Federal DEA controlled drug schedules are available at www.deadiversion.usdoj.gov/
    schedules/schedules
Federal OSHA information is available at www.osha.gov
National Association of Veterinary Technicians in American, www.navta.net
State-specific veterinary OSHA information is available through many of the state
    veterinary medical associations, as well as through the American Veterinary Medical
    Association; links to state veterinary medical associations can be found at www.avma.
    org/statevma

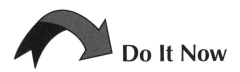 **Do It Now**

Assign one of the doctors in the practice who is a member of the AVMA and the state veterinary medical association with the task of keeping the practice updated with current information on safety and regulations from these organizations. Assign a technician who is a member of NAVTA to do the same.

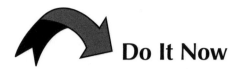 **Do It Now**

Create a corkboard for OSHA, law, and
regulation updates for your practice.
Locate this corkboard in the employee
lounge or break room, or near the
computer or electronic time clock
or main employee entrance.

9

PATIENT RESTRAINT

The animals are the reason we love what we do. Yet they also present challenges when it comes to administering the care and treatment that they need. They do not have the capacity to understand that we are trying to help, particularly when restraint must be applied or uncomfortable measures must be taken to gain a diagnosis or provide treatment. It is the technician's difficult role to be the one who must administer discomfort, in order to provide comfort. Even when the task is not going to be painful, animals must be still and quiet, and the restraint necessary may increase your patient's anxiety and make things worse. Frequently, less restraint is better. Animals tend to resist the restraint more than the treatment or procedure. When that pet's anxiety results in fear or aggression, then the veterinary team must remain safe and keep the animal from hurting itself or others. All of these factors must be taken into consideration as we deliver compassionate care.

What is the best way to put a frightened and/or aggressive patient at ease?

If you know in advance that a fearful or aggressive patient is coming in, you can schedule them a longer appointment time during a less chaotic part of the day. If the patient has been seen by your veterinarian in the past, you may also be able to provide a sedative medication that the client can administer at home prior to the appointment.

Once the patient arrives, have the front office personnel or assistant put the family into an examination room so the pet can become familiar with the surroundings. When you enter the room, pay attention to your own behavior as well as the pet's actions. Animals know when you're afraid of them, and this makes them more afraid or more confident in their aggressive stance. You need to remain calm and confident. When you first meet the animal, spend a few minutes establishing a bond with it. Speak softly, and approach slowly. If the pet seems merely fearful, you can try sitting down at arm's length, facing sideways or with your back to the pet, rather than making direct and possibly intimidating eye contact. Talk to the pet owner and begin collecting history or reviewing the visit, so the pet can see that its owner thinks you're okay. The pet may approach you slowly, or you might try inching closer to it. Always keep an eye on the pet's behavior, since you may be vulnerable if the fear turns to aggression. This method can work well for cats, since they accept people on their own terms and in their own time. If you appear uninterested in them altogether while sitting on the floor, you may end up with a cat in your lap.

For animals that are overly fearful or aggressive from the beginning, another approach will be necessary. It may be possible for you to slip a slip-leash over a dog's head, or borrow the lead from the client if the collar is secure and will not slip off the dog's head. Take the dog for a short walk outside in the hall or through the practice, and use simple commands such as heel, sit, etc. This sometimes helps to redirect the pet's energy and build some trust. Also, it establishes you as an authority figure that the dog needs to obey.

With aggressive cats, many of us are very handy with a towel or blanket. Next time, try spraying it with Feliway, which is a synthetic pheromone designed to reduce stress and anxiety disorders. Most importantly, be patient with your patients. They will sense your anxiety, which will only make the situation more difficult for everyone.

What are some restraint tips to use for cats so you do not get bitten?

As with any patient restraint, confidence is the key to success. If you don't feel confident, ask a colleague to handle the feline patient, and then stand back, watch, and learn. When it's your turn, assess the situation, develop a plan, and do it. Delaying actions and repeating attempts only make it worse for the pet and you. A synthetic calming pheromone such as Feliway can be used to your advantage when sprayed on the towel or bedding.

A perfect approach to removing an aggressive cat from a pet carrier can be unlatching or unscrewing the top. When you lift the lid, have a towel ready to cover the cat and scoop the unsuspecting feline up. Do this quickly, so the cat does not have time to flip and face you or to escape.

Retrieving a cat from a bank of cages can be more difficult. If the cat has flattened itself back into a corner, use a small box or carrier with the door removed to push slowly into the corner, and persuade the cat to enter. Then you can gently but swiftly turn the cage on its end as you cover the open end. The right type of cage can double as an anesthetic induction chamber. Some cats can be lassoed with a slip leash around the neck, and tugged out of the cage opening. Then you can scruff the cat with the other hand as it comes close to the cage door. Once you have a handle on the cat, restrain it further using the typical kitty "stretch" of the scruff and hind legs. Cat restraint bags work for some, but tucking the flailing limbs of a cat, complete with claws at the ends, can be nearly impossible with some cats. Towels work better for containing all of the limbs; you can roll up the patient in what we affectionately call a "kitty burrito." Cat muzzles may work to prevent bites, but they can increase the cat's fear or anger and still leave you with four limbs to subdue. These devices lead you to believe that less is more, and minimal restraint is sometimes the answer. However, safety should always be first. Be careful when finally releasing your patient, because some cats have immediate revenge on their minds! They are also very quick when faced with a threat, so be prepared for them to leap off the table. Doors and windows should be closed, and a towel or blanket should be handy to throw over the cat if needed.

RESOURCES
Animal Handling and Restraint (CD-ROM), by Helen Scott, RVT (Lifelearn 2002)
Animal Restraint for Veterinary Professionals, by C. C. Sheldon, DVM, MS; James Topel, CVT; and Teresa F. Sonsthagen, BS, LVT (Mosby 2006)

How do I get over tension from a dog bite to my face? How can I overcome my fear of getting injured by a patient?

While you should retain a healthy respect for the damage that a patient can inflict, this fear should not interfere with your ability to be comfortable or efficient in your work. If you have experienced a traumatic injury, it is common to feel anxious when faced with the same type of breed or species that inflicted it. You need to realize that it wasn't a personal attack, and the pet was reacting to its heightened emotions of fear or anger. Before you face that same type of disturbing situation or patient again, take a few deep breaths and center your feelings. The animal will react to your fear as well, so it helps you both if you can release those anxious memories.

Be sure you are involving your team members in the restraint of patients. Seek their advice and assistance in difficult situations. If there is a patient you are fearful of handling, request a more experienced or qualified person's help. Watch that person's approach, evaluate his or her success, and have him or her explain the reason he or she chose the method he or she used. Then you can practice the same technique on a stuffed animal or docile patient before advancing to a more difficult patient.

Knowledge is power, and extra training on patient restraint can help you feel more able to handle future patients and avoid injury. Training should also involve topics related to the behavior and body language of animals, which will assist you in reading of patients' behavior. When you come to understand their natural instinct for fight and flight, or lashing out when cornered, you can empathize with animals and approach them from a position of respect. During daily tasks, if you are uncomfortable with a patient's attitude or behavior during a procedure, ask a team member to confirm your assessment and then approach the attending veterinarian regarding medical sedation.

Your job is to provide medical care and treatment of your patients, not to risk your life and limbs performing procedures on dangerous pets. There are times when the veterinarian may have reason to deny medical sedation, in which case you can ask him or her for assistance in restraining his or her patient. Perhaps he or she knows a technique you can learn, or perhaps he or she just does not realize how intense the situation has become.

How do I tactfully inform an owner that his or her animal is aggressive and needs sedation?

Pet owners are afraid for their pets to experience pain and discomfort. They also don't want to feel that they have a "bad" pet, or have been a "bad" pet owner. Explain that the pet is demonstrating anxiety, which is completely natural, so it is the veterinarian's recommendation that the pet receive some minor sedation to provide calming and keep everyone safe, including the patient. Always focus on the best interest of the pet. It may be appropriate to add that the procedure itself is not painful, but the pet needs to be still and the restraint can cause a pet to become anxious or worried and a wrestling match would only make the situation worse.

If you notice the pet becoming more anxious, you can mention it casually at first. You might say something like: "Fluffy is beginning to look a little worried; we may need to discuss some type of sedation when it's time to take the radiographs." This will mentally prepare the client for what might be coming. If sedation is discussed, be sure to explain the medication, process, and recovery so that the client can make an informed decision. Your practice may have the client sign an approval form, so it is important to discuss the potential side effects and dangers of the sedation or anesthesia. The client can feel some measure of control over the situation if he is making a choice to help his pet endure the visit. It may be possible to administer sedation with the client present, so that the client can comfort the pet as the sedative takes effect. This will make the client feel needed and helpful. For pets that demonstrate negative behavior issues on a routine basis or at an extreme level, it may be your practice's policy to gently recommend behavior modification and to provide resources for help. This is usually a conversation that needs to be initiated by the doctor because of the potential sensitive feelings of the client. Ultimately, you want the experience to be a pleasant one for the pet and client.

10

PATIENT HISTORY AND VITALS

A patient's visit to your practice begins with obtaining the patient's baseline vital signs and recent history. Obtaining vital signs such as temperature, weight, and heart and pulse rates can often be a challenge, since patients do not understand that an accurate weight depends on their cooperation, and the rectal probing that often comes with obtaining a temperature can be uncomfortable. Even standing still on a weight scale can be difficult for nervous, excited, or painful patients. A cat that is purring on the examination table may seem content, but his motor makes it difficult to hear the inner tickings of his condition, so you must have a few tricks up your sleeve. Oftentimes, these vital signs are taken in front of the anxious family, so we must also take their emotions and observations into consideration. Every appointment begins with establishing previous history, and this history can be extensive when behavior issues have brought the family to your practice. Beginning the appointment right sets the tone for the rest of the visit that follows.

What are some tricks to obtaining an accurate weight on small or bouncy patients?

It sounds easy enough to get the weight of the patient. Yet this can be complicated by many factors. Typically, the veterinary practice has a floor scale in a public area so that the client can help obtain an accurate weight on a dog, which is helpful. The client can lead his pet onto the scale, or set the pet on the scale and use his hands to help keep the smaller dog in place until the scale zeros out and confirms the accurate weight. When a dog is moving a lot, either trying to escape or just being nervous and shaking, it can take several seconds for this weight to be confirmed. Some dogs are quite fearful of the scale, which feels unstable beneath their paws. It can be helpful to offer a treat; hold it (or have the client hold it) in a closed hand close enough for the dog to smell to maintain the dog's concentration for a few seconds before giving her the treat. If you try this method, always ask permission of the client, since some dogs are on strict diets.

Cats present a different problem, depending on their personality. In most cases, you will want to depend on a pediatric or "baby scale" for obtaining accurate weights on any patient under fifteen pounds, including smaller dogs. Typically, these scales measure weight in ounces, and it is helpful to post a conversion chart on the wall by the scale so that the ounces can be converted to a decimal of a pound. Again, the scale itself will wiggle and feel unstable beneath the pet, and this is quite frightening to some patients. With a small dog, gently laying your hands around or lightly on the pet may help. Cats are notorious for trying to slink off and escape, and the more bold felines may take a flying leap if given the chance. It's important to keep your eye on the patient until the scale levels off, rather than watching the needle. You will not get an accurate weight on a cat that is now under a table! With cats that are highly aggressive, there is another method that can be helpful. Weigh the cat inside his carrier on the floor scale. Safely remove the cat in the examination room or into a cage as the doctor directs. Then weigh the carrier alone, and subtract the two numbers. This is quite accurate, but do note the "cage-plus-cat" weight and then the weight subtracted by the weight of the carrier so that, during future visits, the technician knows this technique was used and is preferable for this feisty patient!

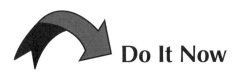 **Do It Now**

Generate a chart for converting ounces to pounds, and post it near the baby scale.

What is the best way for me to obtain an accurate temperature on an unwilling patient?

The gold standard for body temperature is the rectal method. With good restraint, it can generally be obtained even from an unwilling patient. However, the thermometer should give you an accurate reading in a short period of time. Keep in mind that some of the devices that are intended for humans have larger probes than our feline patients may appreciate, so it is best to have several types of rectal thermometers available. The proper equipment needs to be located in every likely area of the hospital. This will save time searching around the facility and making an anxious patient wait.

There may be situations when you need an alternative to the rectal method. Quite often the technician needs to work solo, whether in the exam room with a client watching or treating multiple patients in the treatment area. When using non-rectal thermometers, you need to do a comparison study between readings. On the same patient, obtain several readings from each type of thermometer and compare the results. For example, if you determine that an axillary location or ear thermometer is consistently two degrees lower than the rectal thermometer, apply this adjustment when you are using the ear thermometer on a patient. Also note on the medical record what type of thermometer you used, and develop a code to indicate if the adjustment was applied. This way, when a patient's temperature is taken later that same day or on subsequent visits, you will be able to compare the readings accurately.

A patient's temperature is also affected by the pet's temperament at the time of the reading. For overly nervous or anxious pets, the body core temperature will be elevated. It is important to note the animal's disposition when recording a temperature. It is also advisable to repeat the reading later in the visit or on the same day when the pet has had a chance to normalize its emotions and body temperature. This will help you obtain an accurate temperature, but you will still be faced with unwilling patients. Your preferred methods of restraint can be used while taking a temperature, just as they are when performing any procedure, except that you need to have access to the area for which you are taking a temperature. For canine patients, this typically involves supporting the dog's body under the pelvic area to keep it standing.

Difficult cats can be "stretched" in the common restraint method for access to their bottoms. The patient's tail provides a perfect "handle" for gaining rectal access; those patients without tails tend to be the most challenging, regardless of their personalities!

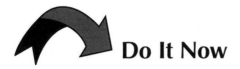 **Do It Now**

Place thermometers in every area of the practice where they might be needed to avoid time-consuming searching, and have more than one type of thermometer available. Mark the thermometers with the name of the area so they are returned when needed.

How do I quiet a purring cat during auscultation?

It is generally thought that cats purr for two reasons: either contentment or anxiety. You will experience patients who are in both emotional states. It's pleasant to have a purring patient that is content and happy to be at the veterinarian's office, and it is easy to feel sympathy for the stressed kitty that is purring despite itself. Yet this little natural motor can make auscultation a challenge. Under the magnification of the stethoscope, the purring is as loud as a freight train as you are trying to count beats and assess heart function. It is handy to know several methods for quieting the train's rumble, if only for a few seconds so you can make an assessment.

Not all cats respond the same way, so you need an assortment of tricks. If you can reach the faucet, running a trickle of water often gets the cat's attention and quiets the roar. When the cat is smelling a treat, the motor also shuts off. You can place a little bit of fragrant cat food in a small prescription bottle in your pocket at the beginning of your shift, and pull it out when you need to examine a feline patient. Another less pleasant smell that is likewise effective is the scent of alcohol. Soak a cotton ball in alcohol, and place it near the cat's nose. The purring will stop as the cat assesses this smelly bit of cotton. For a more hands-on approach, place a finger on one side of the cat's trachea and apply a small amount of pressure. This can work well, and may not scare the cat as much as the water or alcohol methods. Our feline patients are rarely predictable, so have several of these methods handy as you work your way through appointments and treatments.

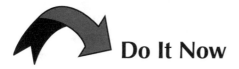 **Do It Now**

Create vials of alcohol-soaked cotton balls
and canned feline diets to keep
in pockets when entering exam rooms
or performing auscultation. Store the food
vials in the refrigerator, and make fresh
vials every few days, or only
create a vial when needed and
discard it at the end of the day.

How can I gather details related to a patient's complicated behavior issues?

Gathering history from a pet owner can be challenging when the patient is experiencing a behavior issue. The technician can help gather information from the family to present the problem thoroughly to the attending veterinarian. A questionnaire should be designed that requires real reflection on the part of the pet owner. Questions should be very specific, but also asked in slightly different ways. Sometimes just rephrasing the question a bit can lead the client to recall a nuance of his pet's behavior that he otherwise forgot. These questions should include what is occurring around the pet at the time the target behavior occurred, who was in the room, the proximity of the pet to other animals or people in the room, and any changes to the pet's environment either in the house or in the neighborhood. Remind the owner that his pet is exposed to specific situations and even areas of the house that most humans do not encounter. The answer could lie in any seemingly insignificant bit of information.

It is helpful, when an appointment is scheduled for a behavior problem, to mail, fax, or e-mail the questionnaire to the client so he can work on it at home. He is more apt to remember the details of his pet's behavior when in his own environment, and he may be able to observe some of this behavior while completing the questionnaire. You can ask the client to videotape the behavior if possible, so there is a visual record of the pet's activities to show the veterinarian.

Another effective method is to ask each family member to fill out individual journals of their interactions with the pet for a week prior to the behavior consultation. All the family members who submit a journal should attend the appointment if possible, because they may have insight to offer the veterinarian. If there is enough lead time before the scheduled appointment, it may be helpful for the client to submit his answers and visual materials prior to the day of the appointment. This way, the veterinarian can review the information and determine how to proceed. Typically, a veterinarian can familiarize herself with a patient visit in the few minutes before the appointment while the technician is obtaining the vital signs. With behavior assessments, however, there is often a large amount of information for the doctor to review, so extra lead time is helpful. These appointment slots may need to be longer as well, and your practice might have a more expensive exam fee set up for these consultations and the time involved to get to the bottom of problem behavior.

RESOURCES
Exam Room Communication (CD-ROM), by Sheila Grosdidier (Lifelearn 2004)
First Steps with Puppies and Kittens: A Practice-Team Approach to Behavior, by Linda
    White (AAHA Press 2009)
Pet Behavior Protocols, by Suzanne Hetts, PhD (AAHA Press 1999)

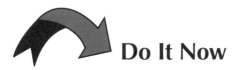 **Do It Now**

Develop a behavior questionnaire for clients to complete with the input of the practicing veterinarians. You can find a sample behavior questionnaire in *First Steps with Puppies and Kittens.*

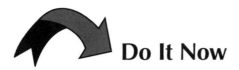 **Do It Now**

Recommend a pet behavior journal for
families to write prior to consultation.
If affordable, have inexpensive notebooks
printed with your practice's name
and logo on the cover to give to clients
for this purpose.

11

PATIENT TREATMENT

We now move into the medical treatment and care of our patients, as they move through various areas in our practices. There are many opportunities for us to help them remain or regain their health and happiness. We have medications available to alleviate symptoms and slow progression of disease and illness. Often the challenge is getting the medication from the bottle, into the patient. There are many routes of administration, and the methods that seem most direct can be the most challenging, such as directly into the mouth of the patient! They have their ways of making it difficult, so we must be armed with just as many tricks up our sleeves. Delivering medication into the ears of our patients can be just as challenging, as they do their best to shake it right back out and onto those of us in the room. When we have questions about medications and everyday medical challenges, we need resources to find answers. Thus, we move beyond the team, past the client out in the lobby, and into the back to tend to our patients.

What is the best way for me to calculate medication doses?

Even when using a calculator to obtain medication doses, an astute technician has the knowledge and experience to determine if the calculation appears to be incorrect. Estimating doses is complicated by the fact that there are some medications that are used frequently, and others that are not. There are situations when we have plenty of time to calculate a dose accurately and recheck our figures, and there are other times when the patient's life is hanging in the balance and we need to get the medication administered, and quick! For frequently used medications, a binder or card file system can be created to refer to, which lists the doses by weight for the medication. Each medication type would be filed under both its generic and brand name(s). This system could include a graduated chart that lists the dose per kilogram. This binder or card file should be easily accessible, with multiple copies throughout the hospital as needed. You can also post edited versions of this material, such as the general mg/kg dose where the medications are actually stored, or you could post simplified charts on the inside of the cabinet door where injectables are located. It is important to update this system as needed when new medications are incorporated into the practice for routine use. Each individual medication chart needs to be easy to read, and the pages need to be sturdy and protected by lamination or sheet protectors.

When emergency medications are needed fast, a large chart of the top handful of drugs that are needed for critical patients can be posted in areas where most critical patients are treated. With a quick glance at the poster, any technician can draw up the appropriate amount of the medication requested by the veterinarian at a moment's notice.

These large charts are helpful for unexpected emergency situations, but for patients that are admitted into the practice that have the potential to crash, you can design a formula spreadsheet that calculates doses of all the emergency drugs for that specific patient's weight. The weight is entered, the formulas are calculated, and then you print out this document and attach it to the patient's cage or treatment sheet. Then, in an emergency, the information specific to that patient is easily accessible. This saves time, and most important of all, it could save a patient's life.

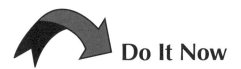 **Do It Now**

Develop one or more of these resources:
general medication dosing charts,
emergency dose chart, or emergency dose
spreadsheet for individual
patient application.

How can I effectively administer medications by mouth (PO)?

For dogs, you can often trick them into taking the medication in a ball of food. Just avoid letting the medication touch the outside of the meat ball so they won't suspect that there is a pill. You can also hide the medication in a dab of peanut butter on the end of a tongue depressor and scrape the mixture onto the top of the dog's mouth. Cats are not so easily tricked, and very few will accept a food treat with or without medication inside while at the veterinary practice. There are also patients that cannot receive food or treats for various reasons. Pill poppers, or pill "guns" as they are sometimes called, can be handy little devices. Caution must be taken not to shove the device too far back into the mouth, as injury can occur. For cats, you have to deliver the pill up and over the hill of the tongue into the small space beyond. Tip the cat's head straight back, apply slight pressure to the lower jaw to open the mouth, and then administer the pill via the pill popper or just drop the pill into the back of his mouth. Gently stroke his neck to encourage the animal to swallow. Once you get the pill in the back of a dog's mouth, you can hold her muzzle closed and blow on her nose. When the dog peeks out her tongue or licks her nose, that is a good indication that she has swallowed the pill.

For smaller patients, you are often delivering small tablets or a half or quarter of a tablet. Put these inside a gelatin capsule that is just big enough for the medication. This is also helpful for delivering multiple pieces of tablets all at once, or for disguising bitter medications. Then, administer a bolus of approximately three milliliters of water into the patient's mouth for a good swallow.

When delivering liquid medication, it is best to place your syringe behind a large canine tooth on the side of the dog or cat's mouth. Deliver the medication slowly, so that the pet can keep swallowing the liquid. For a fractious cat, when you scruff the animal, her mouth naturally comes slightly open, and you can work the syringe or pill popper inside. For a dog, you can use a muzzle that allows access for the syringe or pill popper. Just avoid the teeth!

Are there any good tips for me to administer subcutaneous medications?

When administering a medication that you are not familiar with, ask the attending veterinarian or fellow technician if the medication typically stings or causes discomfort. This will help you prepare for the pet's possible reaction, and can help you choose the needle size and location on the patient to administer the medication. In general, a larger-bore needle will allow you to administer the medication faster, which will make the sting shorter. The poke may be worse, but the pet can get through the procedure more quickly. You can locate the least sensitive area of the patient's body by gently tapping several areas and noticing when you elicit the least reaction. In general, the area over the ribs tends to be more sensitive than the area between the last rib and the hind legs. The dorsolateral region from the neck to the hips is the preferred site for subcutaneous injections. Ask your veterinarian, however, if the drug needs to be administered in a particular location. For example, sometimes vaccinations are consistently given in the same spot on every patient for subsequent tracking of adverse reactions.

As you pull up or "tent" the skin in preparation for the injection, give the area an extra little squeeze just before poking the needle into the area. This helps to alleviate the minor discomfort associated with medications that sting. Use a distraction and move quickly. Dogs can be distracted by patting them on the rump or by someone in the room clapping his hands. You can distract a feline patient by having your restrainer tap the cat on the forehead or nose, or blow on her nose. In cats that show a tendency toward aggression, you can slowly slide them along a tabletop or counter as you administer the medication. They are more worried about the movement than the injection being given. Immediately following the injection, pet the opposite side of the body from where you gave the injection, both as a distraction and to comfort the patient.

What is the easiest method for giving ear medications?

Pets are wary regarding anything that approaches their faces or heads, so good restraint is necessary. If the medication is in the standard dropper bottle, it can be helpful to transfer the liquid to an eye dropper or 1 cc syringe. The syringe allows you to monitor the exact amount of medication being administered, rather than guessing at how many drops you were able to squeeze out from a bottle hidden down in the dark canal of the ear. To make the application as comfortable as possible for the patient, warm the medication to room temperature.

A less direct approach than the bottle or syringe is a saturated cotton ball. Apply the correct amount of medication to the cotton, plus a little extra. Grasp the pinna and pull the ear upward and then back toward the head, to straighten the ear canal as much as possible and allow the medication to reach deep into the canal. While holding the ear up, begin wiping the inside of the ear, slowly squeezing the cotton so that the liquid enters the ear canal gradually. This technique is less of a shock to the patient. The most important tip is to keep holding that ear, while you gently massage the base of the ear for thirty to sixty seconds. This helps the medication go down deep. Then, have a towel handy and pull it over the patient's head quickly while you let go, because the animal will shake! If you're quick and fortunate, the leftover medication along with ear debris will land on the towel as your patient shakes, and not all over you, the pet owner, and the walls of the exam or treatment room. On a small patient who needs both ears treated, you can sometimes keep pressure on the first ear while you repeat the procedure for the second ear, then cover with a towel and let your patient shake. If the pet has debris and discharge in its ears, follow your veterinarian's instructions for cleaning and drying the ear(s) prior to treatment.

What is the best resource to use for learning about medications?

W hen you want to learn more about general medications used in veterinary medicine, many veterinary professionals consult drug formularies such as *Plumbs Veterinary Drug Handbook*. Additional resources are *Saunders Handbook of Veterinary Drugs* and AAHA Press's *Boothe's Formulary*. There are new medications being released constantly for both label and off-label use for veterinary patients. The texts cannot possibly keep up with all of these new arrivals. The best way to discover more about a particular drug is to read the insert that comes along with the medication when it arrives at your facility. These inserts differ from the material safety data sheets (MSDSs) that your practice is required to keep on file. The MSDS explains the hazards and precautions associated with the drug, as well as steps to take if accidental exposure occurs. The drug inserts contain useful pharmacological information, such as the detailed pharmacology, the chemistry makeup of the substance, and exact specifications for dosing and reconstituting. When drugs are put on the shelf for use, these inserts are often misplaced or discarded. Instead, create a binder or organized file for locating these inserts for future reference. Plastic sheet protectors make great sleeves for these inserts, because the inserts are typically long and folded many times over. This file should also contain information regarding the manufacturer and distributor, so they can be called when needed for more details. If you are ever in doubt, the first place to turn is your attending veterinarian. She will have the final word on how you administer any medication to a patient, but you can show initiative by researching some general information on your own.

RESOURCES
Boothe's Small Animal Formulary, by Dawn Merton Boothe, DVM, MS, PhD, DACVIM, DACVCP (AAHA Press 2009)
Fundamentals of Pharmacology for Veterinary Technicians, by Janet Amundson Romich, DVM, MS (Delmar Cengage Learning 2004)
Plumb's Veterinary Drug Handbook, Sixth Edition, by Donald C. Plumb, Pharm. D. (Blackwell Publishing 2008)
Saunders Handbook of Veterinary Drugs, by Mark G. Papich, DVM, MS, DACVCP (Saunders 2006)

What major online resources are available to a veterinary technician for everyday questions on medications, procedures, etc?

Today there is so much information online within the World Wide Web, that this reference source should not be overlooked. You can locate information on medications, procedures, protocols, and general health care. However, caution needs to be used when deciding what information to trust. There are no regulations to govern what can be written on a Web site, so the source of information needs to be scrutinized and approved by your practice's veterinarians. Your practice may also have internal rules about Internet use. If the policy only allows certain Web sites to be accessible, then you may need to seek approval from management to keep a particular Web site from being blocked. Investigate the author of the information, to ensure this person has credentials to substantiate the findings or advice. Look also for other indications that the Web site is reputable, such as veterinary endorsements by the American Veterinary Medication Association (AVMA), American Animal Hospital Association (AAHA), or other familiar organizations in the profession. The national and state veterinary medical association Web sites are helpful and often provide links to other reputable Web sites. Veterinary schools often have university Web sites that contain various topics. The *Merck Veterinary Manual* online is an additional resource. Your practice leaders should be able to direct you to the sources they most trust and want you to refer to when you have questions or simply want to learn more.

RESOURCES
American Veterinary Medical Association, www.avma.org
Directory of links to state veterinary medical associations, www.avma.org/statevma/
    default.asp
The Merck Veterinary Manual online, www.merckvetmanual.com

12

PATIENT SUPPORT

Often, our patients need more support than simply administering a medication by mouth, injection, or dropper. If the pet's health or nutritional state is unbalanced, the pet may need ongoing support via an intravenous catheter. Placing the catheter can be a challenge. Once it is placed, then the challenge becomes preventing the patient from removing or interfering with this plastic lifeline. Newborn puppies and kittens are a special challenge, with ongoing nutritional needs as they grow and develop. They require round-the-clock feedings, which become more difficult as they become older and wigglier. For those patients experiencing breathing or oxygenation issues, the delivery of nasal oxygen can mean life or death for the patient. Yet they have to allow the placement of this nasal oxygen tube and leave it alone once it is placed. Here are some tips on providing this vital support to even our sickest and smallest patients.

What are some tips for me to place a peripheral IV catheter?

The area should be shaved to allow better visualization of the vein, and aseptically prepared with a scrub procedure to minimize infection at the catheter site. It is important to start low on the limb if possible, to allow for additional tries further up if you are not immediately successful. Choose the largest-bore catheter that is appropriate for that size patient, to allow for larger volumes of fluid to be administered more easily. Your restraint assistant will stabilize the pet's movement, but be sure both of you and the patient are in a comfortable position so that slipping and discomfort are minimized. The assistant will occlude the vein to allow for better visualization and access, or a tourniquet can be used instead.

As you try to puncture the vein, you can use the thumb of the hand that is holding the limb to stabilize the vein's movement or "rolling," by placing it alongside the vein. On animals with thick skin, it can be helpful to make a small hole in the skin with the needle first, then place the catheter through this hole. This prevents the barbing of a catheter that can often happen when it is forced through thicker skin. When the catheter is in place, move the thumb and forefinger of the hand that is holding the limb together, and grasp the needle of the catheter, still holding the limb in the same hand. If you hold the needle this way, and the patient pulls his limb away from you, the catheter will not be pulled out. You will continue securing it with the hand that is following the movement of the limb. Remember to indicate to the assistant when to stop occluding the vein, or when to loosen the tourniquet, so that the taping procedure to secure the catheter is less bloody. A technician who has perfected her timing can place the injection cap on the catheter before spilling a drop of blood! The loss of blood itself is not an issue, except that it makes the area messy and cleaning up can disturb the catheter placement. Also, the less blood that stains the pet's fur, the more comfortable the client will be when he sees his pet. Most practices have a preferred method for bandaging catheters, so that the entire team knows how to gain access and remove bandages when necessary.

How can I keep a patient
from chewing on the IV line?

The perfect catheter placement is only as good as the patient wearing the catheter! In the blink of an eye, patients can chew the fluid line, or pull out the catheter altogether. The ripple effect of this one moment in time is wide: The technicians and assistants must take time to replace the setup, patients must endure more restraint, and clients will have to foot the bill for their pets' misbehavior through the cost of additional supplies. There are ways to help prevent this from happening. There are many products that are designed to discourage chewing with a bitter or disgusting taste. These include Bitter Apple and Yuk ointment, and there is a new Vet Wrap product that is advertised as no-chew bandage material. Patients react differently to each of these products, so they may or may not ensure that your catheter is secure.

Close observation of patients is essential. You can also use devices to help prevent access to a limb, such as an Elizabethan collar (E-collar). Even with the collar or "satellite dish" on their heads, pets can gain access to the line that is administering the fluids itself. The line can be relocated by taping it to the E-collar. This prevents patients from getting the line into their mouths. If all else fails, you can apply a muzzle, but patients need to be monitored constantly in an attended location in case the muzzle becomes dislodged or becomes a hazard. Your veterinarian needs to have the final say in using these devices in compromised patients.

What is the best way to feed a neonatal patient?

Puppies and kittens do not always immediately take to a bottle or a feeding, so there are several methods that can be tried with your little hungry patients. The delivery method can vary depending on your preference, your past experience, and the patient's level of acceptance.

Pediatric animal-nursing bottles work well for some patients, and other patients won't take a nipple. You can try using a tuberculin syringe with the needle removed, attached to a teat infusion cannula or shortened red rubber tube. The ideal delivery method allows the milk solution to slowly ooze out the feeding hole when the device is inverted. If the tiny hole in the rubber nipple needs to be enlarged slightly, you can use a hot needle to open it up. The liquid should not come out too fast, however, or the little patient could aspirate. Positioning is very important as well.

You want to simulate the natural nursing position and the warmth of a mother's body. A warmed hot-water bottle can be placed in your lap and covered with a towel. Make sure the temperature is not dangerously warm; this could cause surface burns. With the youngster in your lap, you can use one hand to support the small puppy or kitten's head and entire body, while you stabilize the feeding device with the other hand. On a larger puppy, you may use one hand to support just the head and neck. This hand support allows you to redirect the patient's mouth to the feeding apparatus if the patient is not yet competent at nursing.

Sometimes, older babies get too squirmy to hold safely on your lap. For the wiggly ones, another method involves creating a warm hump on a table to simulate the mother. Put a towel or blanket on a table, and wrap up a warmed fluid bag in another towel to place next to the animal. Use the fluid bag to represent the mother, and prop up the bottle or syringe on it. Do not squeeze the formula out for the puppy or kitten; it needs to actively nurse to avoid aspiration. Do not use this method for puppies or kittens that do not exhibit a sucking reflex.

RESOURCES
Clinical Textbook for Veterinary Technicians, Sixth Edition, by Dennis M. McCurnin, DVM, MS, DACVS; and Joanna M. Bassert, VMD (Elsevier/Saunders 2006)

How do I place a nasal tube for oxygen therapy?

There are several ways in which oxygen therapy can be delivered, including oxygen cages and hoods. Nasal delivery is used quite frequently. The first concern is the patient's comfort, not only to minimize stress but also prevent the animal from jerking away or dislodging the tube while you are placing it, or shortly thereafter. Typically, a local anesthetic such as lidocaine gel, tetracaine, proparacaine, or phenylephrine is applied to one nostril. You should wait thirty seconds for liquids, and five to ten minutes for gels, for the anesthetic to take effect.

A red rubber feeding tube or a clear polypropylene tube is often used to deliver the oxygen. It is important to know the appropriate length of tube for your patient. Measure the tube along the outside of the patient's body from the tip of the nose to the medial canthus. Mark the tube with a piece of tape or marker. The tube will then be fed through the nostril, dorsally and medially, until you reach that mark. You can push the nose pad dorsal-medially while advancing the tube to help avoid the turbinates. Take the remaining tube that is left outside, and flip it over to the other side of the nose or over the head and secure it with skin glue, a staple, or sutures in several places. If a little "flag" of tape is used to mark the stopping point, the flag can be glued to the fur on the edge of the nose to secure it in place close to the entry point. Another tape flag can be applied on the remainder of the tube and glued into place as well, instead of using sutures or gluing the actual tube. It is advisable to put an E-collar on the patient after the tube has been placed to prevent the patient from reaching up and dislodging it with a paw or foreleg.

RESOURCES
Fluid, Electrolyte and Acid-Base Disorders in Small Animal Practice (Fluid Therapy in Small Animal Practice), by Stephen P. DiBartola, DVM, DACVIM (Saunders 2005)
Small Animal Clinical Nutrition, Fourth Edition, by Thatcher, Remillard, Roudebush, and Hand (Mark Morris Institute 2000)

13

DIAGNOSTIC AND
IMAGING PROCEDURES

When our patients arrive for examination, it is often apparent from their physical appearance what might be wrong. Sometimes the diagnosis requires further exploration. When it is suspected that our patients suffer from a cardiac issue, we can use the electrocardiogram to determine their heart function, as long as the patient remains calm and still for the procedure. However, oftentimes the veterinarian needs to look deeper and actually visualize the inside of the patient to gain the diagnosis and prescribe the treatment. Veterinary medicine now has advanced diagnostic equipment to be able to get this inside view of the patient. Radiography allows us to visualize the bony structures, and once we have a good technique chart for our equipment, this is a relatively simple process. Ultrasonography allows visualization of the soft tissues in the abdomen and thorax and helps to define the problem and direct the healing treatment. The technician plays an important role in obtaining results or assisting in the process of using the diagnostic equipment available in veterinary medicine.

What are the best tips when running an ECG on a patient?

Electrocardiography, or ECG, is the process of obtaining a graphic record-ing from the body surface of a patient of the electric current generated by the heart. This diagnostic procedure is used as a means of studying the action of the heart muscle in cases of severe trauma or chronic heart conditions, for example. The heart's rhythm is traced on a paper and/or across a monitor so that it can be visualized and evaluated. The ECG patient should be lying as still as possible, which also requires that the patient be comfortable. Apply appropriate but minimal restraint as needed, and make a soft surface with towels or a blanket for the patient to lie on in right lateral recumbency. The limbs need to be held parallel to each other. Motion needs to be limited, so if the patient is panting or shaking excessively, you can close the mouth and put gentle pressure on the thorax to still the animal. If there continues to be too much movement from the thorax, move the leads distally, but keep them parallel to each other.

When you apply the leads, the order and placement are extremely impor-tant. To remember the correct placement, think of the colors of the lead tips as if you're driving a car: Your right arm stays in the car and does not get tan (so it is white); your left arm rests on the window and gets tan (so it is black); your right foot pushes the gas (so it is green); and the your left foot pushes the brake (so it is red). Apply alcohol or ECG gel to the lead tips to help conductivity. Never use ultrasound gel because this conducts sound waves, not electrical impulses. It is often necessary to monitor the reading you are getting during the procedure, to ensure that the movement of the animal is not causing false readings. Any remaining gel or alcohol should be wiped off the patient before returning the animal to the cage, kennel, or client.

RESOURCES
ECG Manual for the Veterinary Technician, by N. Joel Edwards, DVM, DACVIM (Saunders 1993)

How do I develop a good radiographic technique chart for a traditional or digital system?

Developing a radiographic technique chart is an ongoing process that requires meticulous documentation and continuous adjustment when starting out. It is more a system of recorded trial and error than an exact science, and it will take patience and time to perfect. As you and your colleagues take radiographs during the course of the day, you record the body part being imaged, the measurements of that area, and the setting that was used for the radiograph. You then note how acceptable the resulting image was for that set of data.

As your technique improves and you get closer to knowing the best setting for each circumstance, you eliminate those protocols that did not produce good images. The length of time it takes to create a technique chart will depend on how large your caseload is, and how often your patients require radiographs.

Many practices are entering the realm of digital radiography. Establishing a technique chart for these machines can be less strenuous because the image can be enhanced by the computer if it is underexposed instead of retaken. However, you should adjust your technique as needed for the next similar situation. If possible, you should retake an image until it is correct without computer enhancement. This is easier with a digital system, because you can immediately view and adjust your technique as needed to perform the retake.

You need to avoid overexposure, because the computer cannot adjust this image. The final goal is to complete the process with an accurate technique chart for either type of system. A good tip for reaching this end result is to obtain a patient that is close to its optimal weight. Take survey abdominal and thoracic radiographs until you get the perfect image. From this point, you can determine how to adjust your KvP setting either up or down according to the next patient's size. Repeat this survey procedure for each species of patient that routinely undergoes radiography in your practice.

RESOURCES
Clinical Textbook for Veterinary Technicians, Sixth Edition, by Dennis M. McCurnin, DVM, MS, DACVS; and Joanna M. Bassert, VMD (Elsevier/Saunders 2006)

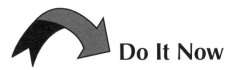 **Do It Now**

Test or develop your radiographic
technique chart using a cat
or dog of optimal size.

Where can I find a resource to learn how to position for good radiographs?

The radiographic image is only as good as the positioning of the patient. You can have the best technique, and be able to visualize every nuance of structure, but if the positioning doesn't aim for the proper place or include enough of the animal's body, the film or image is useless. In most cases, a complete diagnostic study requires two views or images at right angles. When imaging a particular location or lesion, it is imperative to direct the primary beam exactly at this location for maximum visualization and representation of the area. Patient positioning is a combination of skill and the use of good positioning devices such as foam wedges, troughs, and pillows or sandbags. It is also important to have a willing patient that remains still and motionless. For some types of radiographs and many patients, this requires sedation or general anesthesia. Radiographic surveys of the skull or spine require general anesthesia. Even obtaining an image of a limb in a fractious animal can require sedation or chemical restraint. This becomes important from a safety perspective as well, because restraining an unwilling patient can cause harm to the support staff involved as well as to the patient. Beyond these factors, the only way to learn good positioning is to have a great reference book available in the radiology suite, lots of patience, and a doctor who encourages you while you learn how to obtain the best internal view of the patient.

RESOURCES

Atlas of Radiographic Anatomy of the Dog and the Cat, by Horst Schebitz and Helmut Wilkens (W.B. Saunders Co. 2004)

Clinical Textbook for Veterinary Technicians, Sixth Edition, by Dennis M. McCurnin, DVM, MS, DACVS; and Joanna M. Bassert, VMD (Elsevier/Saunders 2006)

Practical Diagnostic Imaging for the Veterinary Technician, by Connie M. Han, RVT; and Cheryl D. Hurd, RVT (Mosby 2004)

Radiography in Veterinary Technology, by Lisa M. Lavin, CVT, BA, MBA (Saunders 2006)

How should I restrain a patient during an ultrasound?

An ultrasound is an imaging process that can take quite some time, depending on the patient, the doctor, and the body parts to be explored. It is important that the patient remain comfortable during this process, so that the best images can be acquired. Often this procedure involves measuring structures or assessing blood flow, or taking digital pictures of structures. You can use some of the same equipment that is used to position for radiographs, such as foam troughs and wedges.

For cardiac ultrasounds, or echocardiography, a special tabletop can be purchased or constructed that allows access underneath the patient's thorax, or to the side that will be down on the table, through holes that are cut out of the top of the table. A blanket or towel on the table helps provide comfort, and a pillow or rolled-up towel under the head helps the patient to stay calm.

Keep the patient calm from the time you remove it from the cage or kennel. Some patients respond well to having their eyes covered during the procedure; most appreciate soothing petting and a quiet voice. It is helpful to explain to the patient what you are about to do, instead of simply grabbing the patient's legs and lying them down on the table. Whether it's the words or the tone of voice, this helps to establish a measure of trust between patient and technician.

14

DENTISTRY AND
DENTAL RADIOGRAPHY

Veterinary medicine has made great strides in educating the pet-owning population as to the importance of good dental hygiene and routine care of the mouth. We see many of our patients on a regular basis for dental cleanings that help to detect current conditions and prevent future problems. Technicians are well equipped to provide this routine care, although the dental cleaning process can be physically demanding on both the patient and the provider, particularly in a practice that performs many cleanings in a single day. The radiographic advances in veterinary medicine are now applied to oral and dental health, although the dental radiography equipment can be quite different to work with and often challenging to position. Advanced dental techniques are now routinely provided by veterinarians and veterinary specialists, and in some states the credentialed technician can assist with these advanced procedures. The challenge is staying current on all of these amazing advancements in veterinary dental health.

How can I make a dental cleaning easier on myself and my patient?

There are various ways to make a dental cleaning easier on both the technician and the patient. Even though your patient is anesthetized, it is important to consider the animal's comfort upon waking. If the patient must maintain an awkward position during the procedure, the animal will awaken stiff and uncomfortable.

Use mouth speculums if needed, but they may not have to be used on every patient. Minimize the length of time their mouths are mechanically stretched open. Place the patient on a cushioned surface such as a blanket or pad, and pad the patient's face and head. To help maintain the pet's body temperature, the surface where the patient lies should ideally be graded so that the water can run out of the patient's mouth and away from the patient's body. Put baby booties on the animal's feet, cover it with another blanket or towel, and dry the patient as you go along to avoid wetness and prevent chilling. If a pet has long facial hair, it's important to move this out of the way. Use small hairclips or bobby pins to move beards and long bangs away so they do not get caught up in the polisher.

In order to make the tartar or calculus easier to crack off, you can flush the mouth with chlorhexidine dental rinse prior to the scaling process. Have a set routine that you follow every time for working your way through the mouth. Clean buccal and labial surfaces, then lingual and palatal surfaces, rinse teeth, then probe, polish in the same order, and flip the patient to repeat on the opposite side. This reduces the number of times you have to reposition the patient on the table or tub grate.

Always disconnect the patient from the anesthesia machine before you reposition, to avoid movement of the endotracheal tube. Minimize movement of the tube during the procedure as well, to avoid tracheal injury. As you move through the mouth, have a sheet of paper or a dental chart for the patient where you can document your findings. Then you can transfer this information to the patient's chart or record. To save time and paper, you can use a small white board as a dental chart for the first draft which you can wipe off and reuse for each patient.

RESOURCES
Canine and Feline Dental Records (AAHA Press 2002)

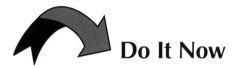 **Do It Now**

Buy a small wet-erase board.
Create a dental chart using this
white board, for use with wet-erase
markers. Transfer information onto
a paper chart after each patient.

How do I position a dog or cat correctly with a dental X-ray unit, and where can I learn better techniques for taking dental radiographs?

Dental radiography is important for diagnosing conditions or disorders of the teeth and oral structures in our patients. Typically, the best method to use in dental radiography is the intraoral technique, where the radiographic film is placed inside the mouth. This positioning of the film helps to minimize the superimposition of teeth and surrounding structures on the area of interest. Correct positioning of the patient is just as important with dental imaging as it is in general radiography, although the equipment is quite different. According to the *Clinical Textbook for Veterinary Technicians,* Sixth Edition, it is easiest to position the dog or cat in sternal recumbency for images of the maxillary dentition, in dorsal recumbency for images of the anterior mandible, and in lateral recumbency for images of the mandibular premolars and molars. You can learn these positioning techniques through several methods, including textbooks, online courses, wet labs at conferences, or in-house seminars by experienced veterinarians or technicians. Contact the manufacturer or distributor of your dental radiology machine to inquire about hands-on learning opportunities, or consult the resources below.

RESOURCES
Clinical Textbook for Veterinary Technicians, Sixth Edition, by Dennis M. McCurnin, DVM, MS, DACVS; and Joanna M. Bassert, VMD (Elsevier/Saunders 2006)
Small Animal Dentistry: A Manual of Techniques, by Cedric Tutt (Wiley-Blackwell 2007)

How do I correct the drift in the arm of a dental radiograph machine?

The dental radiograph machine in general is positioned much closer to the patient than the equipment used in standard radiology. For example, the film focal distance (FFD), basically the distance between the machine and the radiographic film, is only sixteen inches or less for a dental radiograph as compared to a FFD of thirty-six to forty inches in a standard radiograph machine. The other major difference is that, with standard radiography, the unit or machine stays stable and the patient is moved to obtain the best image. In dental radiography, it is the opposite, in that the arm of the dental radiograph machine is flexible and is moved into position over the stable and anesthetized patient. The most challenging part of using this equipment for dental radiography can be the drift or movement inherent in this arm of the machine. You get it set just right, remove your hand, and it magically moves out of place! To counter this frustrating tug-of-war process, maneuver the arm beyond where you actually want it, and then make minor adjustments until the arm is in the right place. You can also let the arm fall where it may, and move the patient's head just slightly to get the proper alignment. The patient is usually a more stable object to reposition slightly and set into place. If the arm is too loose and you need it to have more elasticity to hold it in position, use a large rubber tourniquet around the arm.

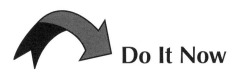 **Do It Now**

Assign a few rubber tourniquets
to the dental radiology machine.
Mark them with white labeling tape
to ensure they return to their designated
place in the radiology suite.

Where can I get training on doing dental blocks for patients needing extractions?

The important thing that sets dental procedures apart from most other elective surgeries is that these dental patients have been coping with chronic pain for quite some time before their condition was discovered and diagnosed. The symptoms typically have to be quite advanced before the pet owner knows to bring the pet in for evaluation. By this time, the patient may be experiencing inadequate nutrition due to painful eating or associated systemic infection, or the pet may be advanced in age so it presents a greater anesthetic risk. In older patients or those that have compromised health, this risk of general anesthesia is a serious consideration to be weighed. The advantages of dental blocks are many. The anesthesia is smoother for the patient, and there is less anesthetic drug required. When the pain is controlled during the procedure, there is less need for postoperative pain medications. There are several techniques for performing dental blocks and a variety of medications that can be utilized. For learning dental blocks and various dental procedures, it is possible to utilize a good reference book or online resources such as the those listed below. These are helpful for learning the physiology and basic theory behind the procedure. However, highly manipulative tasks such as dental blocks are often best learned through hands-on training and subsequent experience. If dentistry is an interest of yours, consider attending a dental conference or watch for major national and regional conferences that provide wet labs on dentistry procedures. Consult the Academy of Veterinary Dental Technicians for further resources. You should consult your state practice act to ensure that technicians can do dental blocks in your state.

RESOURCES
Academy of Veterinary Dental Technicians (AVDT), www.avdt.us
Veterinary Dental Forum, www.veterinarydentalforum.com
Veterinary Dental Techniques for the Small Animal Practitioner, by Steven E. Holmstrom, DVM; Patricia Frost Fitch, DVM; and Edward R. Eisner, DVM (Saunders 2004)
Veterinary Information Network, www.vin.com

15

SURGERY AND ANESTHESIA

When a patient requires surgery, whether it is a minor procedure or a life-saving major surgery, there are numerous considerations that must be addressed. You must document the information in a surgery log to be able to track adverse reactions and cross-reference the controlled substances log to ensure accuracy. To perform the surgery, there are a variety of surgical instruments that can be used depending on the type of surgery. These instruments and supplies need to be properly identified, cleaned, maintained, and sterilized to be ready at a moment's notice. Anesthesia of the patient is a critical element—critical to both the life of the patient and the success of the surgery. The patient's physical condition must be assessed so that the proper anesthetic protocol is used for the pet's needs and the correct procedure is performed. Inhalant anesthesia must be delivered in an effective and safe manner. Although only veterinarians can perform surgery, the technician has a major role in all the other tasks that take place in the surgical suite.

How do I maintain a surgery log properly?

A surgery log can record many types of information and be used for various reasons based on this data. The standard information includes date, client name, patient name, identification number, technician name or initial, surgeon, type of procedure, and start and stop times. Medications are part of this log, including pre-induction, induction, and maintenance anesthesia, including the percentage of oxygen and inhalant anesthetics. When controlled substances are recorded in this log, it allows for cross-reference of the main controlled drug logs and helps find or eliminate mistakes or discrepancies. It is also beneficial to record the patient's level of anesthetic risk, blood work that is performed prior to anesthesia, and any adverse reactions to the anesthesia. Consider additional information, such as the size of the peripheral catheter and endotracheal tube used on the patient. This log can also guide client communication, with a place to document that the pet owner has been given an update after the pet's recovery.

A separate document is used to monitor the individual patient. This will include much of the same information but also track the patient through the procedure. It will document the patient's vital signs at predetermined intervals, as well as fluid rates, medications, and reactions. These records are part of the patient's complete medical history, and, as such, they should be maintained for the length of time indicated by your state law or regulations.

RESOURCES
Anesthesia Assessment and Plan Form (AAHA Press 2003)
Anesthesia Record (AAHA Press 2003)
Minor Surgical/Anesthetic Procedure Sticker (AAHA Press 2005)

What is the best way to organize or identify surgical instruments in a pack?

Every surgical instrument is designed for a specific purpose. Scissors are used to cut, but there are many types of scissors used during surgery for different reasons. While needle holders are designed to hold fast to a suture needle, thumb forceps are used to hold tissue, and hemostatic forceps are used to crush blood vessels instead. As a surgical scrub nurse, the technician needs to be able to identify the requested instrument and its purpose. Anticipating the surgeon's needs during the surgery will greatly enhance the timeliness of the procedure and effectiveness of the surgery schedule. The technician is often the employee responsible for ordering, maintaining, cleaning, and repacking these instruments. Following surgery, you should clean and sometimes comingle surgical instruments, and you should return them to their designated packs for the next sterilization and use. Typically, we wrap large, bulky instruments individually, as we do instruments that are not used frequently. We usually wrap instruments that are used quite often in smaller, handy packs to provide additional instruments during a procedure as needed. We tend to wrap various instruments together in packs if they all are used for a particular procedure. These instruments can be color coded using stretchy colored instrument bands so they will all be returned to their proper pack. You still need to be able to identify each instrument and ensure that the packs are complete and all the proper instruments are back together. Each pack should have a list of all its instruments, either posted inside one of the cabinet doors, or in a binder in the surgery pack room or area. In addition, each instrument should have a corresponding picture, proper name, and general use description. It is helpful for these guides to contain the item name and/or number, and the distributor and/or manufacturer, in case they need to be reordered or replaced.

RESOURCES
Veterinary Instruments and Equipment: A Pocket Guide, by Teresa F. Sonsthagen, BS, LVT (Mosby 2005)

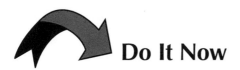

Do It Now

Create a list of each pack's contents, and create a photo guide for each instrument. Locate these lists in a central, easily accessible place.

How much can you safely inflate an endotracheal tube on a dog or cat?

Over-inflation on an endotracheal cuff can cause damage or injury to the patient's trachea, so care must be taken when you're securing an airtight fit for your inhalant anesthesia. Select the most appropriately sized tube for the size of your patient, and do not rely on the cuff alone to provide the extra diameter. Always inflate the cuff to ensure there are no leaks before inserting the tube into the patient's airway. This can give you a rough idea of how much air you may need to deliver once the tube is in place. Then deflate, and entubate the animal. Once the tube is in place in the trachea, inflate the cuff slowly using a syringe while the anesthesia machine is attached to the tube. With the pop-off valve closed, squeeze the reservoir bag to no more than 20 mm/Hg, and listen for leaks around the cuff. You should not hear air escaping or smell anesthetic gases. Repeat this process after the patient has been under anesthesia for several minutes and is more relaxed, since you may need to make an adjustment. There should always be a little bounce back on the inflated ball where you attach the syringe; it should never feel like it will pop if you squeeze it! You can also palpate the trachea, and you should be able to feel the inflated cuff slightly. If you're able to work with an assistant, you can place the syringe on the cuff of the tube and have the other person fill the reservoir bag. As you inflate the cuff, your assistant can tell you how much mm/Hg there is on the anesthesia machine. You should be able to hear air escaping at 15 mm/Hg, and nothing at 20 mm/Hg.

Where can I learn about anesthetic monitoring and anesthesia levels, and the most common anesthetic protocols used for pre-medication, induction, and maintenance?

The concept of balanced anesthesia is now used in veterinary medicine. Whereas in the past a large dose of a single drug was used to anesthetize a patient, whether the drug was inhaled or injected, now anesthesia is accomplished by using smaller doses of a variety of drugs to specifically affect the different components of the anesthetic state. This makes the process safer for the patient, and safer for the veterinary team. General anesthesia is divided into stages that include pre-medication, induction, and maintenance, and these are followed by a recovery period. Various drugs are used to produce each of these stages, dependent on the condition of the patient and the length of the procedure. As new medications are released and studies conducted, anesthetic protocols change and adjust to this progress. Anesthetic monitoring involves monitoring the anesthetic levels that are produced by these medications. The patient's vital signs are monitored every five minutes, and this data is recorded on an appropriate anesthetic record or form. Although there are frequently new advances in monitoring equipment, the use of this equipment does not replace the watchful eye of the technician anesthetist. Ensure that you are staying on the cutting edge of anesthesia by referring to recent sources such as those listed below. Continue to educate yourself on the subject by reading journals and attending lectures and wet labs. You can also consult the Academy of Veterinary Technician Anesthetists (AVTA) for further resources.

RESOURCES
Academy of Veterinary Technician Anesthetists, www.avta-vts.org
Clinical Textbook for Veterinary Technicians, Sixth Edition, by Dennis M. McCurnin, DVM, MS, DACVS; and Joanna M. Bassert, VMD (Elsevier/Saunders 2006)
Clinical Veterinary Advisor: Dogs and Cats, by Etienne Cote, DVM, DACVIM (Mosby 2006)
Lumb and Jones' Veterinary Anesthesia and Analgesia, Fourth Edition, by William J. Tranquilli, DVM, MS, DACVA; John C. Thurmon, DVM, MS, DACVA; and Kurt A.

Grimm, DVM, PhD, DACVA, DACVCP (Wiley-Blackwell 2007)

Small Animal Anesthesia and Analgesia, Third Edition, by Diane McKelvey, BSc, DVM; and K. Wayne Hollingshead, MSc, DVM (C.V. Mosby 2000)

Small Animal Emergency and Critical Care for Veterinary Technicians, Second Edition, by Andrea Battaglia, LVT (Saunders 2007)

Veterinary Anesthesia Update, Second Edition, by Nancy Brock, DVM, DACVA (Nancy Brock 2007)

16

LABORATORY

There are few patients that can be diagnosed without the use of laboratory tests and procedures. The veterinary practice often performs many laboratory tests in-house, as well as maintains a variety of testing procedures that are requested from outside diagnostic laboratories. Oftentimes there are multiple labs that supply the practice with the answers they need. Receiving and interpreting the result are the ultimate conclusions, but before this can happen, the appropriate sample must be collected using the proper method. Then the sample must be processed, the paperwork completed, and the package delivered or picked up by the correct laboratory in a timely fashion. Ultimately, the communication among the team must be smooth to ensure that the sample gets to the laboratory as needed, so the patient can benefit from the information it holds. Finally, there is much to be learned to operate the in-house equipment and produce accurate results. An extensive list of resources is provided to help the veterinary practice team reach the correct diagnoses in order to retain patients' good health or restore their well-being.

How do I improve client compliance in obtaining a fresh fecal sample?

An animal's feces are routinely examined in the veterinary practice for intestinal parasites, ova, blood, and mucous. Depending on the region of the country in which the patient resides and the pet's routine activities or exposure factors, it is recommended that the companion animal have routine fecal examinations at least annually, if not more often. For these routine fecal lab tests, a sample obtained by the pet owner at home is sufficient and won't subject the pet to the dreaded fecal loop. But if the client doesn't bring the sample in, it is difficult to run the needed tests! To improve compliance with clients, send owners home with a prepaid fecal collection jar that has a scoop already attached to the inner lid. This makes the collection easy for the client, and the client is more likely to comply because he has already paid for the test.

An alternative method that is a little more fun is to give the pet owner a Ziplock® bag with a tootsie roll and dog cookie inside. The tootsie roll is to demonstrate the size of the sample needed and becomes a treat for the owner; the dog cookie is the treat for the pet! The Ziploc bag is for transport back to the clinic.

Clients need to be informed that if the samples will not be examined at the veterinary practice for several hours, they need to refrigerate the sample. Feces that will be examined for parasites can remain refrigerated for up to three days.

RESOURCES
Clinical Textbook for Veterinary Technicians, Sixth Edition, by Dennis M. McCurnin, DVM, MS, DACVS; and Joanna M. Bassert, VMD (Elsevier/Saunders 2006)

What is the best way to obtain a fungal culture sample?

The dermatophyte that is commonly called ringworm is a fungus that invades hair and the superficial layers of skin. It can cause areas of chronic, mild inflammation that acquire crusty debris. There can be singular or multiple lesions, and hair loss varies among patients inflicted with ringworm. For example, a cat may show no hair loss at all. This dermatophyte is identified by use of a standard culture medium called Sabouraud's dextrose agar, or a selective medium such as dermatophyte test medium (DTM). A fungal culture can sometimes be a hit-or-miss process, depending on the collection method used to obtain the sample. Pluck hairs from the perimeter of any obvious lesions and collect bits of scale or crust. However, you want to avoid heavy contamination with saprophytic fungi or bacteria which can overgrow in the medium and make ringworm detection difficult. If the lesion is considered to be contaminated, you can gently cleanse the area with 70 percent alcohol. In patients such as cats that are not exhibiting obvious symptoms, use a new clean or sterilized toothbrush and aggressively brush the entire pet from head to tail for two to three minutes, paying particular attention to the face, the feet (especially between toes), and the inside of the ears. The bristles of the brush are then lightly brushed across the surface of the culture plate.

RESOURCES
Clinical Textbook for Veterinary Technicians, Sixth Edition, by Dennis M. McCurnin, DVM, MS, DACVS; and Joanna M. Bassert, VMD (Elsevier/Saunders 2006)
Dane County Humane Society, www.giveshelter.org/sitemgr/ringworm

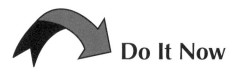 **Do It Now**

Purchase a supply of new toothbrushes in
individual packaging to keep on hand
in the laboratory.

How can we communicate that a sample is in the back to go out to the lab?

The efficiency of an outside laboratory is only as good as the communication within the practice: The sample has to reach the lab in order to produce results! There are many points where communication can break down, so it's critical to design a protocol that keeps all of these steps in mind:

- One person can be in charge of samples each day in a small clinic. In a large clinic, there should be two people assigned and one standby, depending on the shift arrangement. Rotate this responsibility if needed to share the workload.

- The sample is prepared by the attending technician, including necessary laboratory request forms.

- The attending technician phones for a sample pickup, if a routine daily pickup is not already scheduled for that particular laboratory.

- The sample is stored in a well-known and easily visible location, in a clearly marked holding box.

  - For room-temperature samples, a holding box can be located in the in-house lab or receptionist area.
  - For refrigerated and frozen samples, clearly marked plastic should be located in the refrigerator or freezer.

- Create signs using brightly colored index cards: Sample To Go Out In Lab, Sample To Go Out In Refrigerator, Sample To Go Out In Freezer (dry-erase boards can be used as well in each location). The sign also indicates where staff members need to go to find the samples.

  - For samples that will be picked up during the day when the front office is open, the front office staff can be notified that there is a sample to go out with one of these signs.
  - For samples that need to be set out in a lockbox or taken to a drop-off location, these cards can be left in a visible spot for the last technician or receptionist on staff (whoever is assigned).

▸ Maintain a lab checklist; document the samples to go out. Each step of the protocol is initialed and time stamped, and the person who delivers the sample to the pickup driver or lockbox/drop-off box will sign off when this transfer occurs.

The result is a set protocol that everyone can be trained on. It also provides accountability because someone signs off on each step of the process. This way, if there is a problem, the sample can be tracked back through the team members who processed and handled the sample.

RESOURCE LIST FOR THE LABORATORY
Resources for Urinalysis
Handbook of Canine and Feline Urinalysis, by Carl A. Osborne, DVM , PhD; and Jerry B. Stevens, DVM, PhD (University of Minnesota 1981)

A Handbook of Routine Urinalysis, by Sister Laurine Graff (Lippincott Williams & Wilkins 1983)

Interpretation of Canine and Feline Urinalysis, by Dennis J. Chew, DVM, DACVIM; and Stephen P. DiBartola, DVM, DACVIM (The Gloyd Group, Inc. 1998)

Laboratory Procedures for Veterinary Technicians, by Charles Hendrix, DVM, PhD; and Margi Sirois, EdD, MS, RVT (Mosby 2007)

Laboratory Urinalysis and Hematology for the Small Animal Practitioner, by Carolyn A. Sink, MS, MT; and Bernard F. Feldman, DVM (Teton New Media 2004)

Veterinary Technician's Daily Reference Guide: Canine and Feline, by Candyce M. Jack, LVT; Patricia M. Watson, LVT; and Mark S. Donovan, DVM (Wiley-Blackwell 2002)

Resources for Fecal Analysis
Diagnostic Parasitology for Veterinary Technicians, Third Edition, by Charles M. Hendrix, DVM, PhD; and Ed *Robinson, CVT (Mosby 2006)*

Laboratory Procedures for Veterinary Technicians, by Charles Hendrix, DVM, PhD; and Margi Sirois, EdD, MS, RVT (Mosby 2007)

Veterinary Clinical Parasitology, Fifth Edition, by Margaret W. Sloss, DVM, MS; Russell Kemp; and Anne M. Zajac, DVM, PhD (Iowa State Press 1994)

Veterinary Clinical Parasitology, Seventh Edition, by Anne M. Zajac, DVM, PhD; and Gary A. Conboy, DVM, PhD (Blackwell Publishing 2006)

Veterinary Parasitology Reference Manual, by William J. Foreyt (Wiley-Blackwell 2001)

Resources for Hematology
Atlas of Veterinary Hematology: Blood and Bone Marrow of Domestic Animals, by John W. Harvey (Saunders 2001)

Avian and Exotic Animal Hematology and Cytology, by Terry W. Campbell, DVM, PhD; and Christine K. Ellis, DVM (Wiley-Blackwell 2007)

Diagnostic Cytology and Hematology of the Dog and Cat, by Rick L. Cowell, DVM, MS, MRCVS, DACVP; Ronald D. Tyler, DVM, PhD, DACVP, DABT; James H. Meinkoth, DVM, PhD, DACVP; and Dennis B. DeNicola, DVM, PhD, DACVP (Mosby 2007)

Laboratory Procedures for Veterinary Technicians, by Charles Hendrix, DVM, PhD; and Margi Sirois, EdD, MS, RVT (Mosby 2007)

Laboratory Procedures for Veterinary Technicians, by Paul W. Pratt, VMD (Mosby 1997)

Laboratory Urinalysis and Hematology for the Small Animal Practitioner, by Carolyn A.

Sink, MS, MT; and Bernard F. Feldman, DVM (Teton New Media 2004)
Schalm's Veterinary Hematology, Fifth Edition, by Bernard F. Feldman, DVM, *et al.* (Wiley-Blackwell 2000)
Veterinary Hematology and Clinical Chemistry, by Mary Anna Thrall, DVM, MS, DACVP, *et al.* (Wiley-Blackwell 2004)

Resources for Cytology

Avian and Exotic Animal Hematology and Cytology, by Terry W. Campbell, DVM, PhD; and Christine K. Ellis, DVM (Wiley-Blackwell 2007)
Diagnostic Cytology and Hematology of the Dog and Cat, by Rick L. Cowell, DVM, MS, MRCVS, DACVP; Ronald D. Tyler, DVM, PhD, DACVP, DABT; James H. Meinkoth, DVM, PhD, DACVP; and Dennis B. DeNicola, DVM, PhD, DACVP (Mosby 2007)
Laboratory Procedures for Veterinary Technicians, by Charles Hendrix, DVM, PhD; and Margi Sirois, EdD, MS, RVT (Mosby 2007)
Laboratory Procedures for Veterinary Technicians, by Paul W. Pratt, VMD (Mosby 1997)
Veterinary Parasitology Reference Manual, by William J. Foreyt (Wiley-Blackwell 2001)

INDEX